# Happy Feet: A Diary Of A Traveling Histologist

A Healthcare Professional Travel Assignments Experiences
Lorraine Lala B. (ASCP)CM

## Table Of Contents

Acknowledgments iv

Part 1: What Is a Histologist? 1

Part 2: My First Travel Assignment 6

Part 3: My Time in Minnesota 14

Part 4: The Beaver State Called Oregon 21

Part 5: Indiana: The Hoosier State 26

Part 6: Florida: Where I Eventually Became a Grown Up 30

Part 7: It is Not All Peachy in Georgia 35

Part 8: Taking the Gloom Out of Ohio 39

Part 9: A Grueling But Rewarding Job in Pennsylvania 43

Part 10: The World of Surgery in North Carolina 49

Part 11: Quite a Tough Time in Washington State 53

Part 12: Leisurely Trips to Missouri and Washington DC 57

Part 13: New York, New York 66

Part 14: Sunny California 72

Part 15: Aloha, Hawaii 80

Part 16: Me and the Rest of the World 85

Closing 107

Resources

# Acknowledgments

First and foremost, without God, this book wouldn't be possible.

Sometimes for me the only way to discover what I'm supposed to do with life is to try different things until I see what works and what fits right with my heart. I'm indebted to a host of healthcare professionals who have influenced my concepts of histology. Among them are Pathologist Dr. Michael Awasum and hundreds of healthcare agencies that aided me. From the start my skills in becoming a histologist were sharpened by Supervisor Linda's technical expertise. Last, and most important, I want to express my gratitude to several hospitals, which over the past eight years have opened their department doors to me so I can help save lives. This travel journal is dedicated to my family, friends, and co-workers.

Travel begins with stepping - and finding – out

# Part 1

# What Is a Histologist?

I'm a traveling histologist, a job which is hard to define for many. It seems not a lot of people are acquainted with my profession or my world. So before I get into the nitty-gritty of my traveling experiences, let me share some general information about my line of work.

## What is Histology?

When I was still in school, we were taught about words and their origins. Usually, the definition of the term is in the name itself. You simply need to break it down.

For example, the word "science" is from the Latin word "scientia," which then means "knowledge." Science, therefore, is the process of learning something. Here's another example: "technology." It's actually derived from two Greek words, "techne," which means skill or art, and "logia," or logic or learning. Thus, "technology" is the process of applying one's skills to come up tools or machines that are logical solutions to a problem.

It's the same thing with histology. The word comes from combining two Greek terms: "histos" and "logia." It stands for tissues and learning, respectively. Put two and two together, histology therefore is a study or learning about the tissues of the body.

Now you may ask why it's referred to as tissues and not cells or atoms or whatever else the body is made up of. A long time ago, during the early days of science, the brilliant minds behind its growth dealt with tissues of the body.

## What Do Histologists Do?

I'm often asked by friends and family – none of whom have sufficient background in my field – what it is that I do, and if I'm even a doctor. The answer is no, if we're talking about job descriptions, among others. I'm also not a nurse. However, that doesn't mean my job is any way less important. Histologists do play a very critical role in the field of science, in general, and medicine in particular.

One of our primary responsibilities is to help diagnose, treat, and identify diseases and microorganisms such as the viruses and bacteria that cause them. We're able to accomplish this by getting samples, referred to as specimens, from our patients. Hence, we're definitely exposed to biological threats. Most of our time is spent working in laboratories. In school, we're taught how to prepare specimens such as freezing and cutting before they're mounted onto the slides and seen through the microscope or other apparatus. Hence, the job requires a very high degree of precision, hand-eye coordination, and control. Although we're required to work like most of the professionals – that is, only 8 hours a day or 40 hours a week – we're sometimes needed for longer hours, especially when we have many specimens to check.

We also work with blood and anything related to it such as transfusions. First, we have to correctly identify the blood type of the patient and ensure the potential blood for transfusion is the right match. You have no idea what can possibly happen to a patient who receives the wrong blood. It can actually kill them!

Histologists also need to monitor the patient, particularly if he or she is already undergoing treatment. We should be able to tell if the patient is already responding to the medications or not or if there is another kind of treatment that is more ideal for them.

I'm not an oncologist, which has been my earlier aspiration, but I don't mind working as a histologist because I also get to work with cancer. This is because the disease itself can affect tissues and organs, especially if it's already in the later stages. Although we can't prescribe medications or treatments to them, we can work alongside other medical professionals as a team. This allows us all to do something to make our patients well.

It's very important for a histologist to not just know about the machines or equipment, but also to truly understand what they're meant for. With the onset of new technologies, the histologist's role also includes working with computers and other kinds of devices.

## What Opportunities Are Available?

One of the great things about being a histologist is that you do have different opportunities that you can explore. I began as a histologist technician working in one of the largest hospitals in New York. I spent most of my days in the laboratory until I later became a traveling professional (which is really cool).

Like most of the health-related work in the country, the need for histologists is expected to grow to around 14% from 2006 to 2016. This is according to the Bureau of Labor and Statistics. Moreover, while hospitals will still remain to be the biggest employers for histologists, I can already see the increasing demand in diagnostic laboratories and other smaller health care facilities. The demand is also felt in other parts of the world, such as Europe, so if you want to broaden your horizon further, you can try your luck there. Nevertheless, because the requirement may be different from one place to another, you may have to take some certifications before you can work there.

## How Do You Become a Histologist?

One of the first things you to do to become a histologist is work it into your education. As early as possible you need to have a solid foundation in the sciences, including mathematics, and technology, such as computers. You should learn to love your chemistry and biology. Be truly interested in these subjects!

After that, you should proceed with your higher education, such as getting a certificate in histology technology, which is offered by your local college or university. I took a different route and took up a pre-med course, which is still acceptable since the main point here is to gain higher knowledge about biological sciences like anatomy and physiology.

Is it okay to apply for an online course instead? If you're planning to do this, just make sure that the program is accredited by the NAACLS (National Accrediting Agency for Clinical Laboratory Sciences). It's not enough that you're dealing with a legitimate online school because even if it is the program might not be accredited and you will definitely have a very hard time finding work. Your diploma or certificate is not considered valid.

A full histology course can last between 4 and 5 years, after which you earn a bachelor's degree. You can also try to earn the associate degree, which is good for one to two years, but you need to have an experience in the field for at least a year before you can apply for a certification.

## How About Certification?

Although ours can never be considered as a medical license, histologists still have to obtain a state license that we need to renew every three years. One of the things to remember is that this license is different among states. There is no such thing as a national license. Hence, you need to make sure that yours can be accepted if you are planning to move to another. If not, take its licensure exam. So far, based on experience, it's not as difficult as you would like to think, especially if you're already working in the field. Your experience and knowledge can help you breeze through every exam. The certification, by the way, is provided and approved by the American Society for Clinical Pathology. Histologists are also certified by a board called the ASCP and this certification is accepted by all states.

There are two types of exams provided, depending on your exact job description. These are histotechnologist and histotechnician. The main difference between the two is that the former is seen as more advanced. Simply put, your skills and knowledge on anything related to tissues are much higher since you are tasked to perform more complex procedures and techniques. You will also be working with more pieces of equipment. The good thing is you can move up the ladder and become a lab supervisor or even its director. You can also teach in universities or colleges.

## Are We Paid Well?

For me, income is relative. Sometimes, you're paid less than the other professions, but you don't end up living paycheck to paycheck since you are good at controlling your expenses. I know of many people who earn a lot, yet struggle to make repayments to their utilities and credit cards because they prefer to spend the money on the less essential things of life.

To answer the question, the salary of a histological technician varies from state to state. Definitely, you're paid more if you become a histology technologist. That is aside from the other benefits provided by the laboratory or the hospital. If you get the chance to work in more established labs or facilities, you can get more benefits such as a 401(k), paid vacation leaves, performance bonuses, and other incentives. Your continuing education may also be paid partly or even in full by your employer.

The rates and benefits, nevertheless, can vary from state to state. New York may pay higher than Texas, but you also have to consider the cost of living, wherein NYC is more expensive than the latter.

I have travelled on assignments for many years, taking thousands of photographs either en-route, or at my fantastic destinations. I have chosen a few which I have special memories of and which I hope you will also enjoy.

# Part 2

# My First Travel Assignment

# The Phone Call that Changed my Life

Phone calls are never created equally. There may be one from your mother reminding you to take your lunch and go home early for a nice family dinner for her home-cooked meals. I also received calls regularly from my colleagues whenever there is trouble or important information they needed to retrieve from me.

However, the phone call I received on August 2006, while I was working as a cytotechnologist prep technician in New York, is by far the most special. It is one that brought me to different places both inside and outside the United States that I've always dreamed about. It was indeed the call that ultimately changed the course of my life.

To understand me really well, you have to know that I was born in Jamaica and my family moved to the United States when I was very young. Back in Jamaica, my parents had to toil every day, sometimes including nights, to send all of us to school. I can see them break their backs and sometimes, embrace their crushing spirits for a dream that wasn't theirs. They were fighting for mine.

Thus, I grew up with one thing in mind: I have to work hard and do my best in school. For somebody who is actually a nobody, I can only do so much. To excel in education was the only option I had.

# Creating the Dream

I had a wonderful childhood in Jamaica, but it wasn't enough even for me.

For me, Jamaica is one of the most beautiful places in the world. It's laid-back and time seems to pass by slowly, so we really didn't feel most of life's pressures. Our home was only a few meters away from the beach, so when I needed to take a breather and clear my head, I gave in to the call of the waves and sand. With some book in hand, I'd sit on the powdery sands for hours until the sun began to set. Then, I'd wait for the small shacks and beachside restaurants to turn on their lights — a way of ushering the positive vibrations of the night.

When time permitted, I'd grab my makeshift surf board and tried my luck in the waves. However, my parents decided to leave the country and search for better opportunities. As a young child, I can remember boarding a plane going somewhere I had only heard of – United States of America. Without really knowing, what's out there for me, I knew that US meant better life.

## The Conversation with the Counselor

New York wasn't really easy for me and my family as the city was completely different from where I came from. It demanded more from all of us: more work hours, more money, and more time for something else other than the family. However, we believed in its promise of equality and diversity, that it's what we needed if we truly wanted to make something out of our lives.

I spent high school in New York and later, took up university in Virginia, where I took pre-med. Before I joined the university, I was privileged to be able to talk to a career counselor. After taking a short examination — it's supposed to help decide the best career for me, he said — I sat down nervous yet excited to know what the result was.

Mr. Counselor then said, "looking at your results, it seems you are better off in a career related to science. Have you thought about becoming a nurse or a doctor?"

"Actually, sir, I did, but I wanted to do something different. I was thinking maybe I can be an oncologist. I've always been interested in anything related to cancer."

"That's good news. Who knows we may need more oncologists in this country or perhaps in the world. We've practically seen the steady but very quick rise of cancer cases in the United States. But, you should work hard as it will be very grueling for you. You have to be ready to spend many hours of study. But then again, I'm quite confident that you will make it seeing how you seem to be doing very well in the sciences."

I could not have been happier. It's one of the best affirmations I had received in my life. I was becoming more confident of the career that I wanted to pursue. After a few minutes of more discussion with the counselor, I thanked him for his help and time then bid goodbye.

## Working as Cytotech Prep

To become an oncologist takes many years of education and I was very much aware of that. To help me ensure that I can certainly reach my goal, I took up pre-med as my university course. I labored very hard and worked as much as I could with my education so I could get good grades and be one of the best students in school.

Right after graduation, I worked a few jobs until I was given a chance to move back to New York and work in a major hospital as a cytotechnologist prep technician.

Being a cytotechnologist prep technician isn't really close to being an oncologist, but the concepts and methodologies are still very similar. I still get to work with specimens and worked with cancer-related cases, such as melanoma. As a technician, I was one of the staff in the clinic in charge of preparing specimens, covering slides, and double-checking every tissue that entered the laboratory. It was paid quite well, but more than the salary, I was so inspired by working alongside our country's pathologists and cytotechnologists. I surely took the opportunity to learn as much as I can from their methods, work ethics, skills, and knowledge.

*"This is it!" I told myself. "This is the career I wanted to pursue for myself. It's not far out from my pre-med course, it allows me to work with specimens and help in the treatment of people including cancer patients and it's something I definitely love doing."* I thought I was already set for life on this.

I was wrong.

## Histology Found Me

It was summer of August 2006. The heat was sweltering, but my mind was so troubled, I didn't even realize then that it was summer. Truth be told, I loved my job since it's close to what I truly wanted, yet I longed for something else — an adventure, a major challenge. And I wanted to be a real doctor. I wanted it so bad, that I started praying earnestly. The desire then became so strong one day that after saying my prayer at work, I wrote my resignation letter even when there's no other job in sight. God and the universe certainly worked in mysterious ways. The next day, while at work, with my letter in hand ready for submission and with doubt in my mind, my phone rang, reflecting an unknown or private number. First, I ignored it. It wasn't really my habit to entertain calls from strangers. Yet it was persistent, so I thought that maybe whoever was on the other line truly wanted to talk to me.

When I picked it up, the person introduced herself as Nancy. She said she was working for an agency. She talked a little about the company she's in, then shared the best news I'd heard in my entire life.

"We are looking for histologists who wish to travel. We came upon your name when we asked for references and we're wondering if you're interested in the position."

Without any doubt in my mind, I answered a resounding yes. What a golden opportunity for me! This job meant so many things, including becoming a histologist — and a traveling professional at that. It's very rare to hear such type of position in the industry. I truly felt honored to be chosen.

What made the deal even sweeter was the long list of benefits I will enjoy. These were medical and dental insurance, 401(k) plan, liability insurance, per diem and weekly pay, paid holidays, car rental, and vacation leave. I can even choose my own home! Best of all, the company can help in continuing education.

Of course, I had to go through a grueling process before I can enjoy the rewards and be able to travel. I was interviewed by some of the managers in the company I would be working for, and they had to perform an in-depth background check. Fortunately, I passed all of them. After they took care of everything, I was ready to go.

## I Fell in Love with Arizona

In less than two months, I moved from the urban jungle that is New York to the vast desert lands of Arizona, where I was supposed to work in a derm facility. I didn't know much about the state, so I decided to do some research and found out it's a Midwestern state. The climate is said to be desert, so it has a milder winter than other parts of the country and humid summers. Can't complain as winters in New York can be very horrendous. It's the kind of climate change that I liked. Besides, it reminded me of Jamaica.

Arizona, however, is a very huge state. It ranks 6th among all 50 states and places 33rd when it comes to population. In 2013, more than six million people lived here.

I worked at a derm facility with a quite easy work shift, which began at 4:00 p.m. and ended at 12:30 a.m. I was frightened since I didn't know what to expect on my first day, but the facility was ready for me. The manager walked me through the entire facility, acquainting me with the protocols, equipment, and people as we went from one section to the other. My colleagues were all very warm, courteous, and friendly. It then became easy for me to blend in and be comfortable with my brand-new job and brand-new life.

For the next 13 weeks, I handled as many cases as I could. These include different skin diseases and melanomas. I was in charge of removing the affected tissue from the patient for processing. I marked the specimens correctly and used grossing ink. I was doing more than technical work. I had to perform at my best since other people's lives were at stake.

## Exploring the Beautiful Arizona

Lab work required only 40 hours per week from me. This meant that weekends were free! Cost of living here was lower than New York's and it's more relaxed as well, so I had the time and money to explore it.

Arizona was incredible.

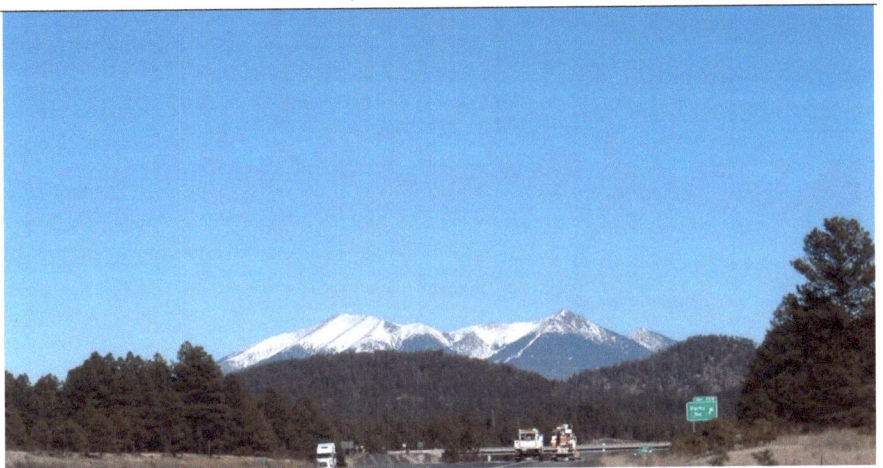

I can't believe that I never took the time to travel this far. Perhaps, I let my prejudice control my mind, believing it had nothing to offer other than the desert sand and the Grand Canyon. For months that I stayed here, I still felt I hadn't seen everything.

On my first weekend, my lab friends took me to a thrilling trail experience in the Grand Canyon. We arrived in Flagstaff and rode a free shuttle that took us to the bottom of the canyon. After we paid the fees, we were then off. There are a lot of trails to choose from, but since it was my first time to do something like this, we opted for the easiest way.

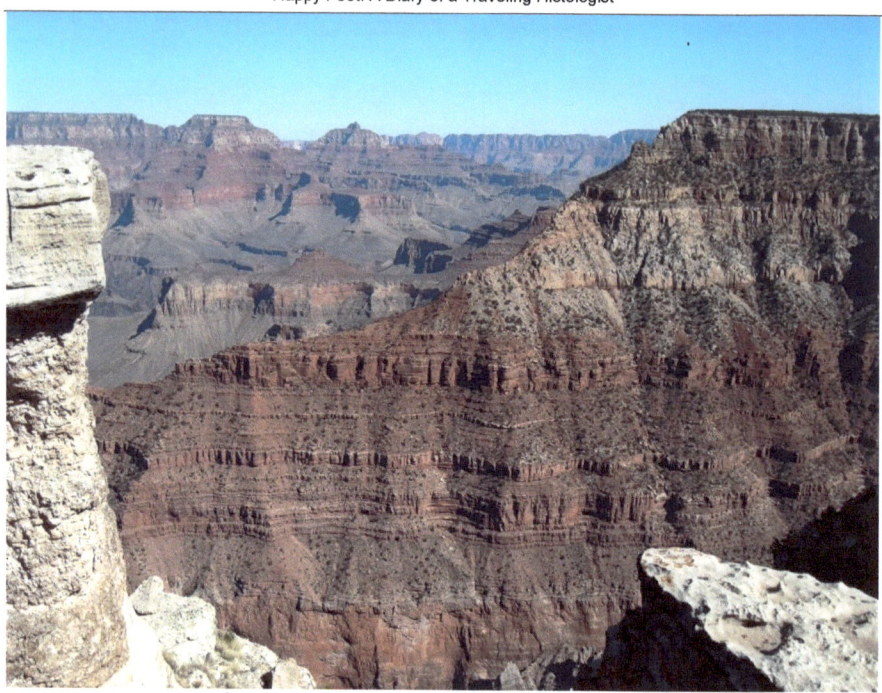

All nice words pale in comparison to the beauty and majesty of the Grand Canyon. The massive red boulders and land formations, the cliffs, the natural sounds, the people — I felt I was just transported to a whole new dimension or universe. It may sound sci-fi, but that's exactly what I felt. It took a whole day for us to complete the trail, and even then it seemed we saw only a small fraction of the huge park! I vowed myself that I'll be back.

When I heard about the "ghost towns of Arizona," I could not let go of the chance to experience them. I did some research and discovered that there were many of them! I chose Goldfield Ghost Town on North Mammoth Mine Road in Apache Junction. Set during the 1890s, it obtained its name from the gold mines within the area. It was definitely a prosperous time, especially for the miners who settled here to take advantage of the precious ores. However, prices eventually dropped, affecting the small town's economy. Although it tried to rebuild itself a couple of times, it eventually died sometime in the 1920s.

Nevertheless, it left us saloons, blacksmith shops, breweries, schoolhouse, and a meat market, just to name a few. There were also a bordello, a railroad, and entrances to the mines. To further attract us visitors, cowboys were all around. When I went there, I actually felt like I was in the movies.

Interestingly, despite being called desert, food was incredibly abundant here. I especially loved Midwestern food such as Tex-Mex, perhaps because I grew up on barbecue parties among friends and family even when I was still in Jamaica. There are many great restaurants in the state such as the Mission, Shinbay, Kai, and Talavera. I walked through vast vineyards and hung out in wine cellars, as well as visited comedy bars and clubs with open mic nights. I even played in one of the casinos operated by an Indian reservation.

It's amazing how everything can work out well for someone. If I hadn't answered the call or said yes to the agent, I would not have experienced this. I'm happy I took a leap of faith, trusted my instinct, and opened my mind to awesome possibilities.

# Part 3

# My Time in Minnesota

I had a great time in Arizona and I definitely gained a lot of awesome friends that I will treasure forever. However, it seemed I was called to do something else, so later I moved to another state, this time Minnesota.

## A Short History

Minnesota is considered to be one of the northernmost states in the United States because it already shares a border with two provinces of Canada; Ontario, and Manitoba. That's why it's referred to as the North Star State, amongst other nicknames, which you will learn about later on.

It has a total land area of more than 85,000 square miles with a total population of over five million, making it one of the 25 densest states in the country.

The history of Minnesota is actually very long. You can trace its early beginnings during the last years of the ice age, which explains the presence of very interesting fossils in the state. Before the official arrival of the Europeans, the land was already occupied by the Indians. They had traveled more than 500 miles to get to the state. When they arrived, they made use of the holy quarries using the pipestone derived from them to make their special pipes that were used during ceremonies.

There are also many pieces of evidence that point out how people lived back then: in rock caves. They had used their space to create carvings and other writings on the rock walls, leaving its future generation with something to use to learn about their previous lifestyle. As Indians, they buried their loved ones in mounds, and the state has many of them.

By the 1600s, the fur traders from France arrived in Minnesota, establishing business relations with the Indians. The problem for the Indians started, however, when they dealt with the U.S. government, which needed more land. In 1858, Minnesota officially became the 32nd state of the United States.

The Indians struggled, especially during the Dakota conflict, which drove most of them away from the state. During the 1830s, more foreigners came from Europe, Canada, and the other states. These included Finnish, Yugoslavians, and Italians. Then people of African descent and Mexicans found their way into the state. Today, it's already a mixture of different cultures and traditions, which somehow makes the state very interesting for someone who craves for diversity and new experience like me.

## The Land of 10,000 Lakes

As mentioned, Minnesota, which has St. Paul as its capital, is known by many different names. The most popular is the Land of 10,000 lakes. You may end up asking, "are there really that many lakes in the state?" The answer is a resounding yes! In fact, to be accurate, there are more than 11,000 of them that span more than 10 acres! How amazing is that? These lakes vary in terms of size and depth. For example, when it comes to depth, Lake Superior tops the list with a total depth of more than a thousand feet. The others are around 200 to 100 feet. You also have shallow waters at only 18 feet, which is Lake Upper Red. When it comes to size, the Red Lake, which is divided into Lower and Upper, has a total combined land area of more than 285,000 acres. This is followed by Mille Lacs Lake at around 130,000 acres. Lakes are practically everywhere, there are only three counties that don't have natural lakes.

Lakes are not the only bodies of water that you can find in Minnesota, though. Their natural streams and rivers cover almost 70,000 miles while wetlands are about 10 million acres.

I would say that Minnesota is a perfect contradiction to Arizona, which is more arid since it's surrounded by desert. It's a breath of fresh air, actually, though because of its location, winters can also be a bit harsh. Sometimes it gets too cold. I wish I were in Arizona!

## The Gopher State

The Gopher State is a very interesting name for Minnesota. You know, every state in the United States needs to have its "official" flower, hymn or song, or animal. This simply means Minnesota needed to come up with its own, especially since it was already an official state by the 1800s.

Choosing the gopher, however, was not that easy since the animal had to fight the title with the beaver, which were abundant in the streams. The people of Minnesota, especially its leaders and proponents, needed to prove each other's point. In the long run, the gopher received more publicity, and thus, the state became known by such name. This also explains why during my first few weeks in the state, I made an effort to see a real gopher.

## What Was I Doing?

I've been talking a lot about Minnesota in my earliest paragraphs that you may already be thinking, "so what is she doing there anyway?" I didn't go there to have a vacation. I also had to work.

Before, when I was in New York, I worked in a very large hospital, in a comprehensive laboratory dealing with all types of tissue-related cases like those from cancer patients.

Later, when I arrived in Arizona, it was a completely different facility, since it was more related to dermatology.

When I arrived in Minnesota, I also did something else. I went back to the hospital setting, but this time it was already a VA hospital. As such, all of our patients are veterans. It was also my first time to work in a government-funded and –run facility.

As one of the histology staff in the hospital, I worked closely with the veterans particularly those who are suffering from prostate issues. The prostate is a man's organ that is found enclosing the urethra, so it sits very close to the bladder. The job of the urethra is twofold, and one of these is the production of semen, particularly during ejaculation. Semen isn't all sperm. It also has some fluid that is derived from the prostate.

A lot of men think that only the older men develop issues with prostate. The statistics are farther from the truth. Men who are under 50 years old of age can develop prostate problems, the most common of which is called prostatitis, which is the inflammation or the irritation of the prostate. Since it is inflamed, a person develops flu-like symptoms and feels a burning sensation around his sexual organ, especially when he is urinating.

Nevertheless, most of the patients in the VA are over 50, and a good number of them already suffered from more severe issues like prostate cancer. To help us detect and diagnose the disease, we had to perform a core needle biopsy. In this process, we used a special needle to extract a sample suspicious tissue directly from the prostate.

Working with the veterans was a very humbling experience. These are people who at one point offered their lives for the safety of the country, and yet in front of me, they were at our mercy and care. I made sure that I always left them feel that they were properly taken care of.

Anyway, one of the most memorable things that happened to me in Minnesota, career-wise, is that it was here where I witnessed my very first autopsy. This is one of the things that I consider most enriching experiences of my career.

## A Tour around Minnesota

I was fortunate to be able to work only on daytime, so I got to enjoy proper rest in the evening. During weekends and on my paid leaves, I also took the chance to see a lot of attractions, the state has to offer. Two of the most memorable ones were the Crater Lake and Mall of America.

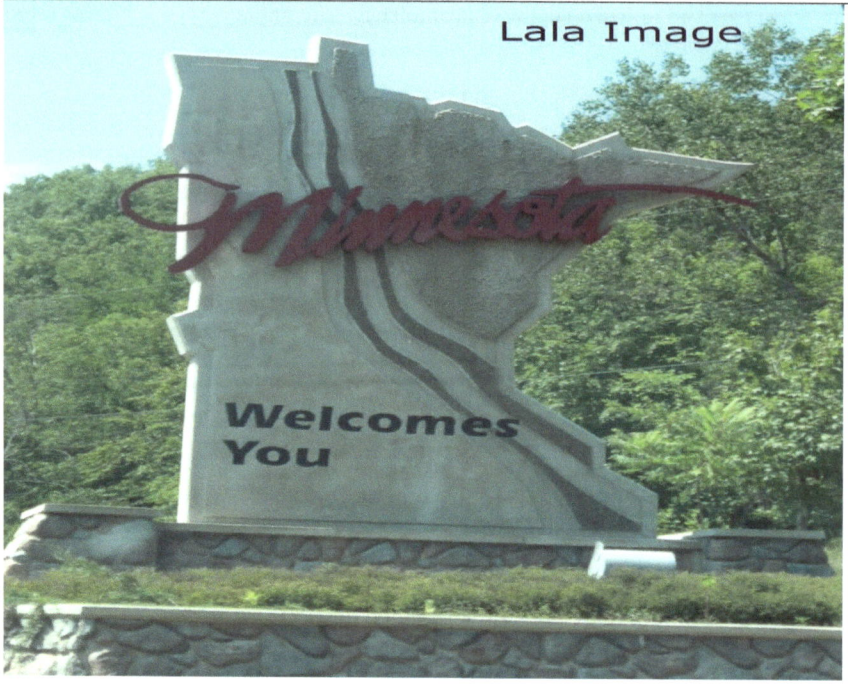

Mall of America, certainly, deserves its name because it's incredibly huge. In fact, I had to be there more than four times, and even then I don't know if I had seen everything of it. It was definitely overwhelming considering I was not totally new to large malls, having spent some time in New York.

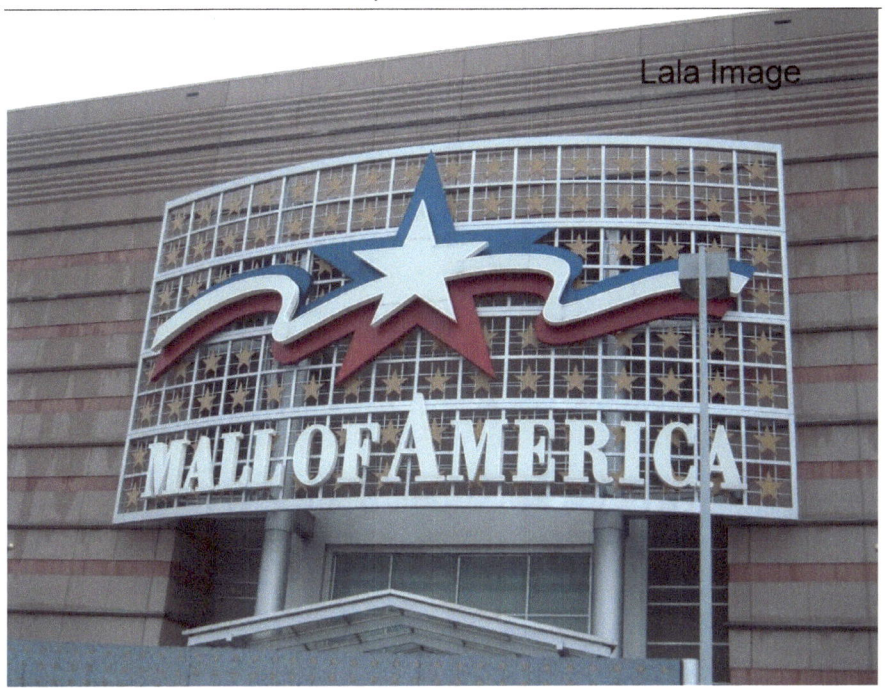

Of course, I went shopping here, but more than that, I explored its many attractions. Some of the most popular ones are the Nickelodeon Universe, Minnesota Aquarium, Flight Simulation Center, and different exhibitions. I enjoyed lunches and dinners in Crave, Buffalo Wild Wings (which I think serves the best buffalo wings I've ever tasted in my entire life), Kokomo's Island Café, and Nordstrom.

I also took some time to visit the Crater Lake.

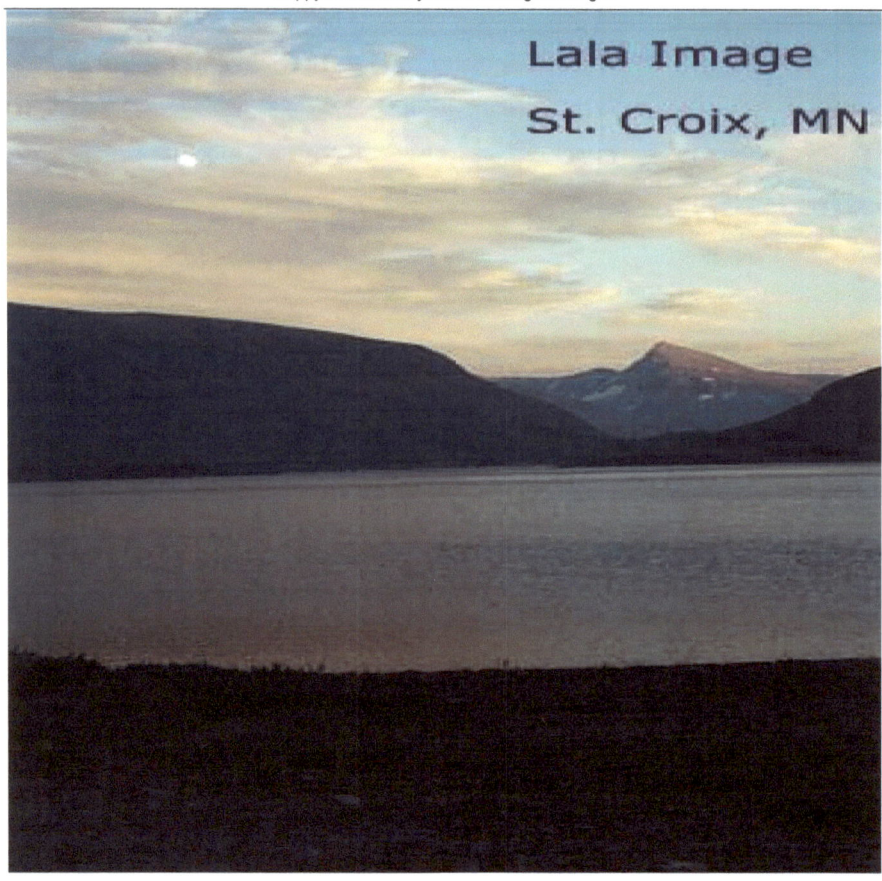

# Part 4

# The Beaver State
# Called Oregon

As a traveling histologist, I have always moved to another health care facility in another state. From Minnesota, I was asked to render my services in Oregon.

Oregon is completely different from the first two states I've gone to (traveling, in fact, has made me realize that even if the country is made up of 50 states, each offers something unique and beautiful). While Arizona is usually arid with mild winters and Minnesota gets quite cold during the fall, Oregon has a perfect mixture of different climate patterns. One, it is close to the Pacific Ocean, so it is normally dry during the summer and wet when fall and winter come along. Then, the higher region can also get very cold that it's almost alpine. It's a great state with a very intriguing climate depending on where you are as of the moment.

Oregon is one of the largest states in America; it ranks ninth among the 50 states. It covers more than 95,000 square miles and has a total population of 3 million, which means it's actually less populated than Minnesota, which has a smaller land area than Oregon. Its capital is Salem.

## A Bit of History

It has already become my custom to learn something about the state's history even before I arrive there. For me, history is a huge part of any place's evolution and culture. It's like me: although, I grew up in the States, I was born in Jamaica to Jamaican parents. What I look like, what I do, and the things I believe in are also influenced by my own history.

Anyway, the initial inhabitants of the state can be traced back to around 15,000 years ago, and just like most of the states within this region, the area was populated by the Indians. During the 1700s, most of the residents came from different Native American tribes such as Molalla, Nez Perce, Umpqua, and Bannock. However, accounts of exploration of the Europeans go back to as far as the 1500s. One of the plausible explanations why they didn't settle here until many years later is that they just didn't take the time to fully explore the land. The Pioneers arrived in Oregon sometime in the 1800s with John Jacob Astor leading them.

One of the most common wrong perceptions people have about Oregon, especially for those who haven't fully visited the United States or set foot in the country, is the belief that Salem, Oregon, was the site of the infamous witch hunt trials. They were actually held in Massachusetts. In fact, the state is called the Witch City! Oregon became a U.S. state in 1859.

## Nicknames!

Like Minnesota, Oregon is also called by its many nicknames. If you can refer to the previous chapter, we talked about the debate Minnesotans had about their official state animal. It was a choice between a beaver and a gopher. While Minnesota chose the gopher, those in Oregon went for the beaver. It is such a beloved animal that it can be found in the state's flag. You may ask, though, what's with the beaver?

First, the animal has played a critical role in the economic growth of the state. Fur hats became more popular because of them, and the number of trappers increased for a certain period of time. Many also like the special "traits" of the beaver, which includes being intelligent, skillful, and ingenious.

Hence of course, being the Beaver State is not the only name the state is associated with. It's also known as the Web Foot State. If you can recall, certain parts of Oregon can have a lot of sunshine than the others. Well, they may also have more rain. Those found in the western area can experience up to 180 inches of precipitation rain in a year. That's definitely a lot of water.

## My Stay in a Nonprofit Hospital

I have been assigned to Oregon to work for a nonprofit hospital. This means that it is being operated mainly for the benefit of the health and well-being of the patients. I am definitely not saying that the other health care facilities don't do that. I am so blessed to have worked with people and businesses that have great compassion for the sick and the needy. So what makes the nonprofits different is the fact that they don't have to please any stakeholders. Thus, their decisions are largely driven by the needs of the patients rather than their economic value. It's a large facility because we offered our services not only to those who are in Oregon but also to patients living in California. The southern part of Oregon, which is where the facility can be found, is close to the northern region of the state of California.

I still continued working as a histology technician, and I was very good at it. That doesn't mean, however, I was no longer challenged. Because of the wider demographics of our patients who are living in two large states, we had to process a variety of tissues every day. Sometimes, I felt that I could not find time to rest, let alone breathe, anymore. Moreover, since it's a nonprofit organization, the services were offered for a very minimal fee, which is used to cover for the expenses of running the facility. The cheaper cost further drove patients to go here.

The truth is that I couldn't complain. Aside from being able to do the work that I love, and I also got to meet very helpful and great people who were my colleagues. They were very unassuming and accommodating, especially for someone like me who had just arrived at the state. Since I worked during the day, I still found some time to enjoy and relax at night with them. They were excellent companions and friends. I had learnt to be so close to them that I am still in contact with most of them.

## Many Sights to See

Surely, I didn't waste time to visit and see different parts of Oregon while I was there. One of the most memorable experiences I had was going to Mount Hood, which is famous for its many trails. We took The Sandy Range trail, since we wanted to explore the outdoors not hiking but biking. I was so glad that this trail offered a path for beginners, so I got to spend more time enjoying the view rather than trying to find my balance. One day, my friends also took me to Clackamas River, which also had a trail laden with incredibly beautiful flowers and greeneries. It made me want to sing the theme song of the *Sound of Music*.

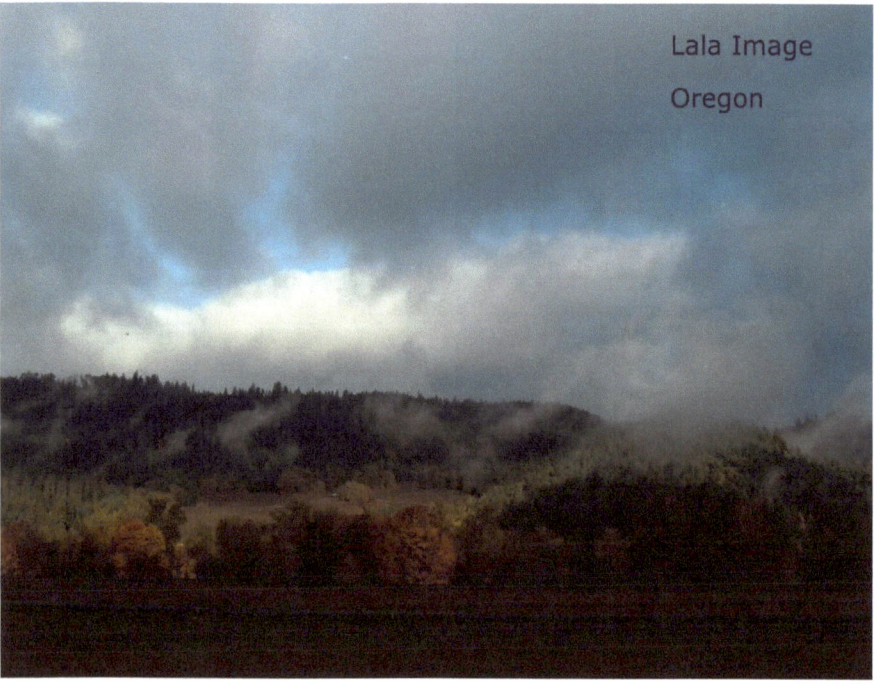

Lala Image

Oregon

I am also so fortunate to be able to see the Crater Lake, which the Oregonians are extremely proud of. Once I got there, I wasn't so surprised anymore. It was truly a sight to behold. It is considered to be the deepest lake in the United States and one of the deepest all over the world. There is good news about it. Since it's a national park, there were days when access to it was free! However, since this area also snows, there are only a few months when you can see the lake in all its glory, with crystal-clear but blue waters.

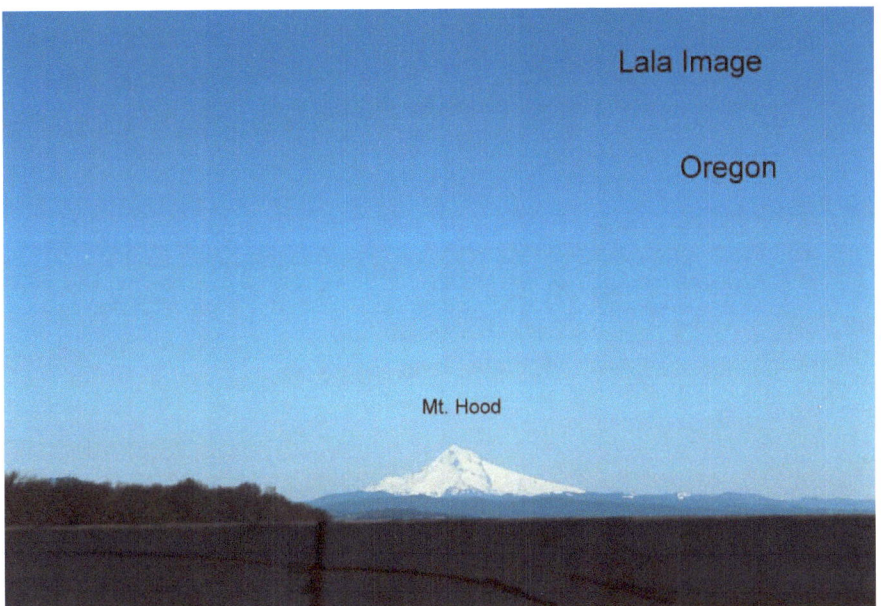

# Part 5

# Indiana: Hoosier State

As much as I love New York and although, I consider it as my home, I had to say good-bye to it for a while so that I can continue to fulfill my job, experience something new, and open more doors of opportunity for myself. Since I was young, I thought traveling would be a great chance for me to discover more about my profession and even, more about my personal life.

From New York, I decided to accept a job in Indiana. If you're wondering why it's called Indiana, it's actually a reference to the Indians that lived and thrived here for many years (a friend once corrected me about the term "Indians)". For him, he preferred calling them Native Americans since even before immigrants and colonizers from Europe came, they had already settled here. They were just called Indians simply because these Europeans thought America is already India)!

These Native Americans played a very large role in the history of the state and the way people lived that many believed it's why it's called the Hoosier State.

Based on my research, there's no definite story behind the word other than a reference to a poem written by John Finley called "the Hoosier's Nest." It was widely read around the time, and people started associating the word with Indiana, although, they didn't truly know its exact meaning. Perhaps it just sort of got stuck.

One thing is for sure, though: it isn't such a large state. Measuring around 36,000 square miles, it ranks 38th among 50 states. However, it has a total population of more than six million, which means it can get pretty crowded in here. As for its climate, I actually loved it, since everything just seemed all right. For example, during the winter, the weather can get cold, but not as much as my experience in New York. On the other hand, during summers, the weather may be humid, but definitely Arizona was much hotter.

Although the state is associated with the Native Americans, their population has drastically been reduced. The state now is dominated by white Americans, which make up around 86% of the entire population.


## Tough Work

Now, you may be interested to know what I was doing there. Well, again, it's a completely different experience from my previous histology-related jobs. In Indiana, I was asked to work with various facilities and diagnostic labs, performing a wide range of tests and services. Indiana has a lot of these labs and health care facilities that sometimes I get too exhausted from traveling. It was also a huge challenge since I was assigned in night shifts. In my previous line of work, I worked in day shifts. I had to reprogram by body clock just to ensure that I can sustain my nighttime work. I also could not count anymore the number of coffee cups I drank.

Nevertheless, this wasn't really a non-issue for me because I loved my work. By the time I was working in Indiana, I had already gained many technical skills. What I needed to develop were my soft skills, such as my ability to work in teams and communicate. Since my job compelled me to work hand in hand not just with my own team but also with others, I was able to enhance the mentioned soft skills. I felt that I became friendlier and became more open to new learning. My job even got me more excited about my profession.

## Seeing Indiana

One of the reasons why I love my job is because I can always include sightseeing during my stay. When I was in Indiana, I did a lot of those. Most of my local friends took me to different adventures. I have to say that these places were a breath of fresh air since most of the things I got to see when I was in New York were mostly man-made.

During my first week in the state, my friends opted to take me to Brookville Lake. It was the hunting season, so I got to experience firsthand how it was to hear gunfire and eat hunted meat during a camp. In spite of that, I was more thrilled with fishing in the lake and exploring the surroundings by taking on the easy trails.

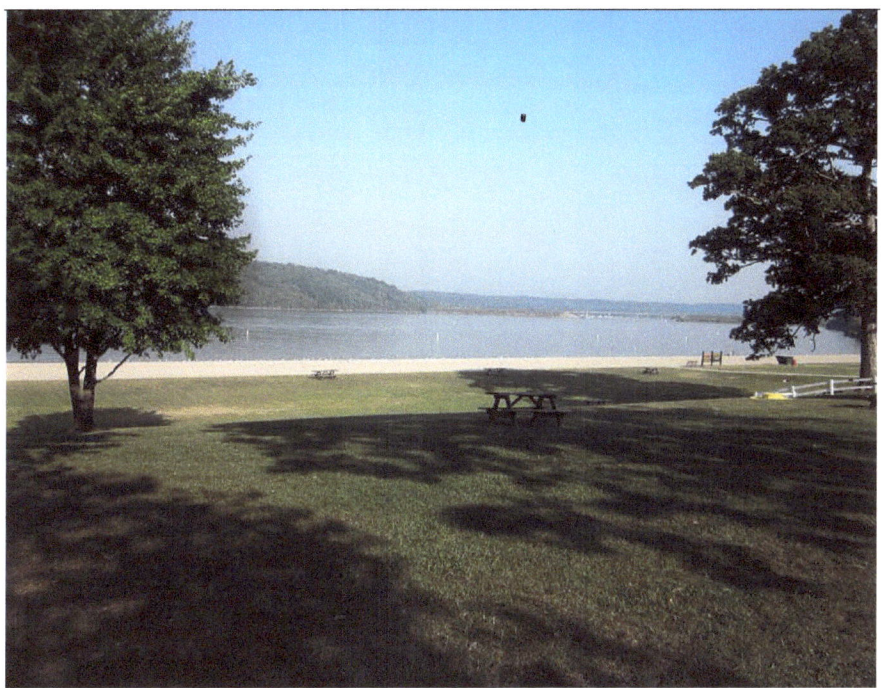

I also loved my time in Fort Harrison State Park, which was one of the closest outdoor destinations for me. Once in a while, I would send gifts and special surprises to my family, and usually that meant checking out the flea markets and bazaars. You would be surprised as to how many kinds of antiques you can find on the street! The people were lovely as well as they normally allowed me to haggle for the prices. At times, too, music festivals and concerts were held here for free. I just bought a few glasses of beers or my friends brought along a picnic basket and sat on the lawn to listen to really cool music.

I also took the time to participate in some of its famous tours such as the Catacombs Tours. In truth, it's not really a catacomb per se. Rather; it's a reference to a once-historic building hidden underneath the now-popular City Market. I am referring to the Tomlinson Hall, a glorious gathering place that was burnt down in 1958.

The Colonel Jones Home gave me a better idea about the Civil War. Open all year round, the home used to be owned by William Jones, a close friend of President Abraham Lincoln, whose house is also nearby. It's a beautifully restored home set to give tourists a glimpse of the life and tension during the Civil War. Indiana is just filled with so much history, culture, and nature that I learnt more from here about life and about my country than when I was still in school.

# Part 6

# Florida: Where I Eventually Became a Grown-up

During the course of my travels, I realized one very important thing: not all places are created equal. Granted, each state offers something different from all the others. They have their own charm that draws you to them, and they also have their disadvantages that allow other states to shine. Yet there are also places that teach you more than their geography, history, and culture. Your stay there has enriched your life in ways that you can never possibly imagine they help you grow up some more. This was Florida for me.

From Indiana, I moved to Florida. I worked in a facility where I dealt with cancerous tumors. That sounds creepy - or morbid - to some, but remember when I told you that I wanted to be an oncologist? This was the fulfillment of that dream. I may still not be in oncology, but I was right into the same circle. There's something about cancer that made it so fascinating to me. Perhaps it's because real cures still remained elusive. I hope that I can contribute to find the real breakthroughs that we need. I am also aware that cancer is a very serious and fatal disease, and its effects to the patient and his or her family go beyond the physical. This is my way of helping them out.

Anyway, I was still assigned in the evenings, but I didn't really have a fixed schedule. That's all right, though, since by now I already had quite adjusted to working at nighttime. While daytime shifts afforded me the chance to take quick trips or visits to attractions, night work permitted me to fully concentrate on the tasks at hand.

I was supposed to work for only three months as was my experience in the other states, but this one lasted for a year! Thus, Florida had somehow become my home. I definitely forged a great friendship and married myself to the job.

The work was also very demanding. The facility expected me to function to my fullest capacity – that means I should be able to work fast and efficiently. I also learnt to be more independent and at times rely on my own judgment or decision - making skill. I have to say that this was one of the hardest jobs that I had ever done, but it was all worth it. It taught me so many things about perseverance, dedication, and passion. I was able to tell myself that truly I was fit to do this job.

## The Many Things that made Florida Memorable

One of the many things that I can never forget about Florida was its climate. It was sunny most of the time, which was just what I needed after spending quite some time in New York. I know how winter can turn for the worse. So the beaches in Florida were such a welcome treat.

Florida isn't really such a big state — spanning around 67,000 square miles, it ranks 22nd in terms of land size — but it is densely populated with people from almost all types of culture. I just think that these families were attracted to the beautiful climate, excellent standard of living, and a wide array of activities you can do here.

Florida is very near to Gulf of Mexico and it has the longest coastline in the country. In other words, it is defined by its beaches. When I had some free time, especially when it lasted for a couple of days, I took some time to hit the beaches of Pensacola, West Palm, and of course Miami. Sometimes I did my quick holiday trips with friends, other times I was by myself. Whether I was alone or not, however, I managed to have such a fantastic time. After all, I spent a portion of my life in Jamaica, where the beaches were also accessible. I felt being surrounded by water will never be uncomfortable or unsecure.

In Miami, I also visited a couple of parks and recreation such as Flamingo Park, which had more than 15 tennis courts to choose from. From time to time I dabbled into the sport. Up on Collins Avenue, meanwhile, is Northshore Bandshell. Miami also has a special program called Art in Public Spaces, which for me was very innovative and daring because it cultivated a sense of creativity and appreciation of the arts to both locals and tourists — that art can happen anytime and anywhere, even outside galleries and museums.

I was also given a time to travel to Fort Myers where I was able to watch games in City of Palms Park and Alico Arena. I think anyone who arrived in Fort Myers should find time to see the famous Edison & Ford Winter Estates. If you're wondering why it's called as such, it's because during winters, the 20-acre plot of land with old but well-tended gardens and equally historic homes used to be a retreat to two famous people in the world: Henry Ford and Thomas Edison. Walking around here, therefore, is experiencing almost the same thing these two people did. One of the highlights will be the botanical garden and the research lab of Edison.

Beachcombing has also become a favorite pastime when I was at the beach, but as much as possible, I didn't bring these seashells back home. After all, they weren't meant to be with me — they're intended to be right here at the beaches.

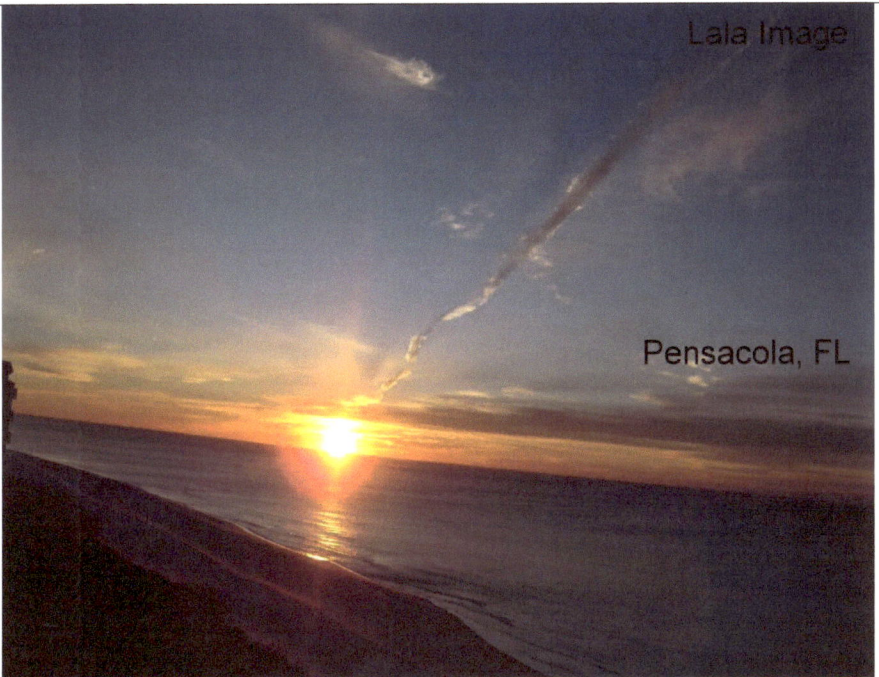

Lala Image

Pensacola, FL

I also visited Pensacola and enjoyed my stay in Johnson Beach. Unlike most of the beaches in Miami or even in Pensacola, this one was quite secluded, but it's just what I needed since it's not yet too commercial. I soaked in history as well as I visited their famous historical village, Saenger Theater, and Fort Barrancas.

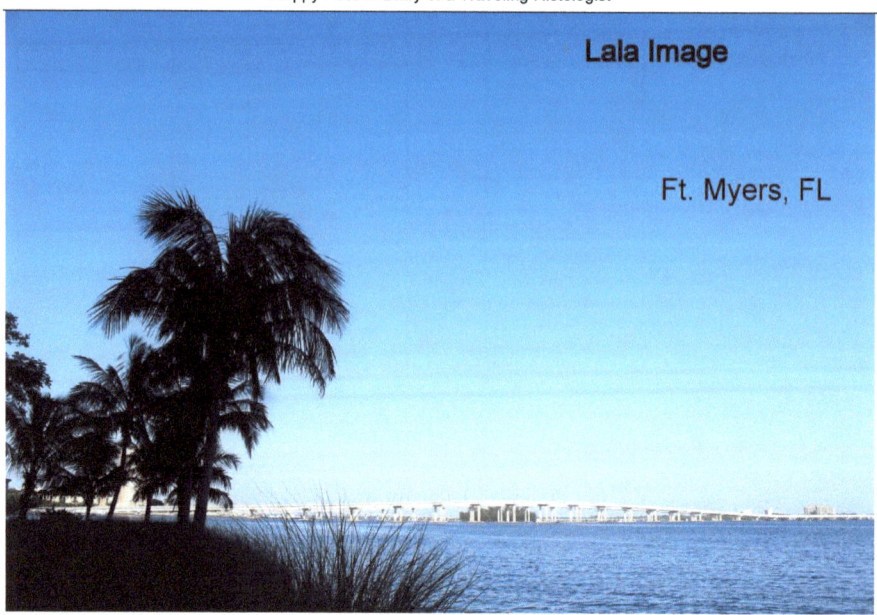

In the winter, the population would swell in the state as snowbirds come, appreciating Florida's warmer temperatures. It is also a great time to catch the Red Sox in spring training- they usually begin in December — at JetBlue Park.

Florida was so kind to me that when I left, it was truly bittersweet. I can't wait to be given the opportunity again to come back to my other home.

# Part 7

# It Is Not All Peachy in Georgia

Before you start misinterpreting my title, let me begin by sharing with you my life as a histologist in Georgia. I have worked with some of the biggest hospitals, diagnostic labs, and other health care facilities all around the country. I have also collaborated with some of the best surgeons and other health care professionals.

In Georgia, it was another opportunity for me to learn a lot in my field since I was asked to work in a hospital that is affiliated to an Ivy League university. For any histologist who has only a few years in the industry, that is certainly a good way to validate my workmanship and ethics.

As it is a large prominent hospital, I always knew that my job was not going to be very easy. In fact, I have already prepared myself for that. What I did not anticipate were two things: transport and inside politics.

I had a huge problem with my commute mainly because of traffic. Rush hour can be horrendous that I got stuck in the buses or taxis for almost an hour. I was so close to getting my own bike, but I did not think it was practical then. It was a good thing that later I worked at night shifts. Rush hours in greater Atlanta are from 7:00 a.m. – to - 9:00 a.m., then 4:00 p.m. – to - 7:00 p.m.

I can effectively deal with traffic. The one thing I was having a hard time with was inside politics. Do not get me wrong. It is not as if there was no such issue in my previous jobs. I always believe that as long as you are working in an industry where you get to meet all types of people, inside politics is bound to happen. Yet what happened in Atlanta, Georgia, was just beyond me. It was so obvious that I did not enjoy my work a lot. It did not matter that I spent most of my time in the lab. Gossip can still find its way there. I met some good friends in the hospital, but I preferred to distance myself so I did not have to get involved in all the drama.

I am not sure why it happened. I guess it had something to do with the aggressive competition among the staff. I mean, it's an Ivy League affiliated hospital, and being given a great position can help create a glowing résumé. For all that I wasn't in Georgia to compete —I was there to do my work the best way I can. I just concentrated on what I was doing, and before I knew it, 13 weeks were over. Thank God, my duty wasn't extended.

## All Is Not So Bad

My job in Georgia was more stressful than usual that my weekends were spent outside my temporary home and into exploring what the city can offer. I wasn't disappointed, thankfully. Minus the traffic, Georgia is a very beautiful state. It isn't like Florida and New York, two of my favorite states, but it has its own character, which I really like.

Georgia, by the way, is very close to North Carolina and Florida. It has a total land area of more than 55,000 square miles, making it the 24th largest state. It has a population density of 165 per square mile; there are more than nine million people living here, making it one of the 10 most populous states. The state's official name is the Peach State, simply because there are many growers of peaches in the area. The state is also widely known as the best source of this fruit.

Some people mistakenly believe that the state was named after George Washington. There's only one state to bear the former president's name, and that's Washington. Georgia is a tribute to the former king of Great Britain, King George II.

There are many awesome attractions all around Georgia, but Atlanta was more than enough to satiate my need to explore. One of the incredible things I'd seen was the Living Walls. It's a very unique art concept. Dubbed as the biggest gallery in the city, it's artwork in public spaces. Simply put, artists use buildings as their canvases, and these are not graffiti at all. Rather, they uplifted the dreary surroundings with eye-popping colors and subjects. This also means that some of the best artworks in the city are for free!

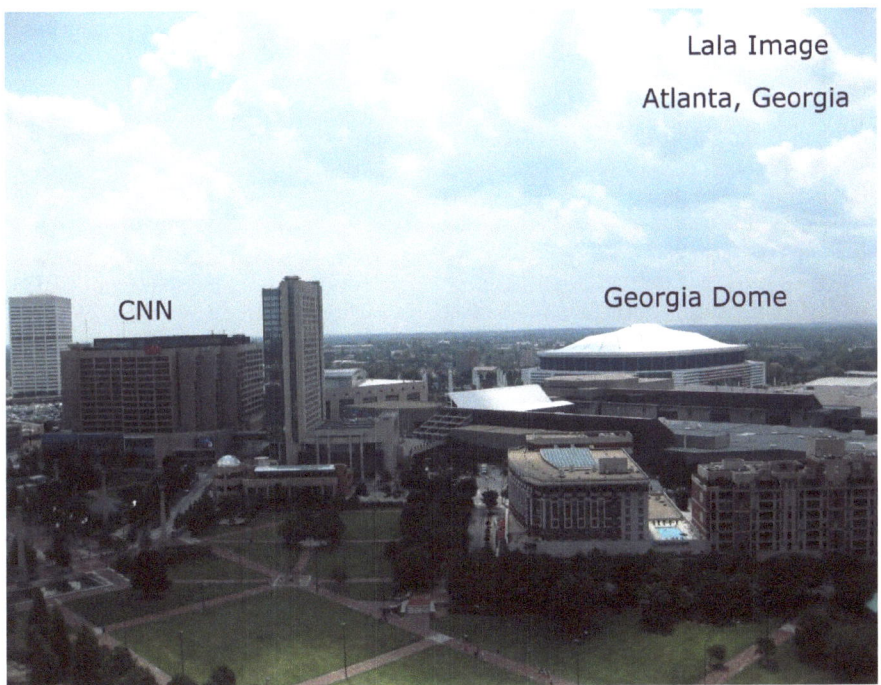

Lala Image

Atlanta, Georgia

CNN

Georgia Dome

37

Twice, I visited Oakland Cemetery for a moment of reflection or for enjoyment. It is a massive garden cemetery with designs inspired by the Victorian Era. From what I've heard amongst the locals, the cemetery has capitalized on that by encouraging visitors to don on Victorian costumes. I think that's a very good dare. You can just take in nature or go to Potter's Field, where you can spread a blanket and have a nice picnic.

I toured Emory University and never failed to drop by the famous Michael C. Carlos Museum. What made it very different from all the other museums I've gone to was that most of its displays were East Asia in origin, such as, from Greece and Egypt.

Moreover, since *Gone with the Wind* was my mom's all-time favorite movie, I went to the house of Margaret Mitchell. Already considered as a historic site and listed in the National Register, the apartment was inspired by Tudor-style architecture. Mitchell lived in apartment 1, with her husband.

Truthfully, you'll be able to appreciate the tour more if you know its significance — that is, it's where she wrote the Pulitzer-winning novel *Gone with the Wind*, which was later transformed into a movie.

I toured the Fernbank Museum of Natural History, rode a bike in the Velodrome, tried Six Flags Over Georgia, shopped at Atlantic Station, watched people played hooky in Piedmont Park, and dined in some of the coolest restaurants and bars in Midtown.

Although I am not really a huge fan of Coca-Cola, I still had a fabulous time in the World of Coca-Cola. Their exhibits were well thought out and visually entertaining, and their movies in 4D theater were surely awesome. I also didn't let go of the chance to visit the CNN Headquarters and to be in awe at one of the biggest public aquariums in the world, the Georgia Aquarium. And when my contract ended and I had to go back home for a bit, I had one last interesting Atlanta experience: Hartsfield-Jackson Atlanta International Airport. What people are saying is really true. This airport can be crazy when it comes to tourist departures and arrivals. I've never seen a real sea of people in my lifetime.

Despite all the trouble and issues I dealt with when I was in Georgia, I can still say it gave me a very memorable and pleasant experience. It helped me grow as a person and taught me how to be truly professional in my line of work.

# Part 8

# Taking the Gloom
Out of Ohio

After a year, my job and life in Florida ended. It was quite incredibly painful for me since I've come to love the sunny state and I knew right away that I was going to miss my friends and my equally awesome job.

Nevertheless, I guess it's pretty normal for any traveler to fall in love and be attached in some of the places he or she gets to visit. In the end, it's always who you are — that is, a traveler — that counts more, and this is what it is for me. It's this type of explanation that encouraged me to move on and instead be grateful for the awesome memories in Florida.

After a year, the agency assigned me to work in Ohio, which was more than a thousand miles from Florida. I knew then that it's going to be yet another new experience for me.

This time, I worked in a faith-based nonprofit hospital. Working at nights, I tackled the laboratory, processing different types of specimens from the many patients we were helping.

My work in Ohio opened my eyes to something more profound and humbling. Being born in Jamaica and spending my first few years there, I definitely had some experience when it comes to faith and religion. My parents also brought the family to believe in God and it was that belief which I carried on with me everywhere I go.

I know that not everyone shares my belief - and that's fine. I respect each person's opinion and argument, but after finding myself in this hospital, I saw how faith can be so important for the entire health care community including the patients and professionals such as doctors, nurses, and, of course, histologists. Many patients with terminal illnesses hung on to their faith as their main source of strength, so you can see them at peace within themselves. You know that they were still hoping for a miracle — that what they have is just a serious disease that can be treated with medications; that the right cure will eventually come along or they're wishing that they are not sick after all! — but they also had some quiet resignation and grace of acceptance. For me, doing this takes more courage than going through a lot of the treatments.

Adding to the somber moments was the changing seasonal pattern of the state. There were really times when everything around me was, well, gloomy: overcast skies, strong outpour of rain, people walking about with pensive moods, as if they were buried in their own thoughts. I am a very cheerful person with a sunny disposition, so being in this situation definitely took some getting used to.

## A Great Tour around Ohio Cities

In order to uplift my mood and inspire me, it became more important for me to take some days off and simply explore Ohio. The state, by the way, ranks 34th in terms of land size among other states in mainland USA; but it's also densely populated. Not everyone appreciates a state with plenty of people, but I do. I just love to interact with people or even simply observing them.

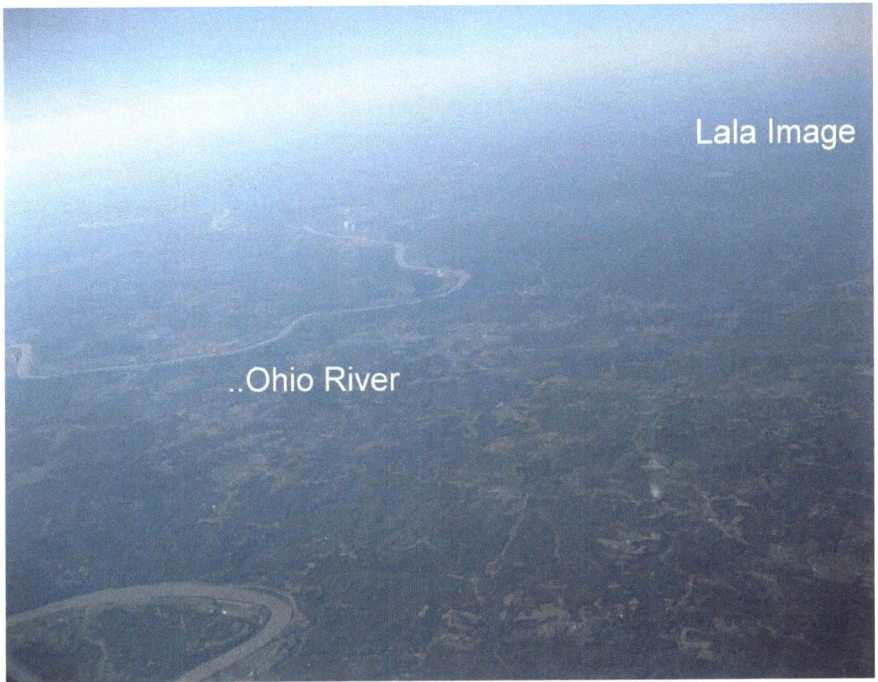

Ohio is known as a Buckeye State, in reference to how the Native Americans called those seeds with deer - like eyes on their skin. Speaking of Native Americans, they were an incredibly large population of them here a lot of years ago. Today, some had just disappeared, while other tribes had assimilated with the rest of the eclectic population.
So far, I conquered three large cities in Ohio. These were Dayton, Cincinnati, and Kettering.

Dayton was perhaps one of my favorite cities in all the places I had visited so far. It offered a wide range of activities! Whether you're looking for history, nature, or entertainment, Ohio can offer you exactly what you want. I think every visitor, who gets to be in Dayton, should visit the Sun Village where some of the Native Americans used to live. The actual village they lived in was long gone, but the people behind the attraction recreated it and added more elements such as performances, rituals, and other activities. When I was there, I met some descendants of Native Americans, and it was so touching to learn that being there was a way of getting back to their roots. I also checked out the National Museum of the U.S. Air Force and the museum that was dedicated to the Wright Brothers. Yup, the city is the birthplace of the airplane.

When I spent a weekend in Cincinnati, I was amazed by the intricate classical architecture of the buildings, many of which were built during the 19th century such as the Music Hall, which had been restored a couple of times and still remained usable. There's also the Art Museum, which houses thousands of art pieces, both potteries and paintings from famous artists.

When my friend suggested that we should visit their cemetery, I was quite hesitant. First, I had the tendency to freak out with anything related to death. Second, it's a cemetery — after all, what can I possibly see there besides epitaphs and tombstones? Yet my tendency to say yes to what I perceived as new experience and adventure got the better of me, and I'm glad I did because the place was just so beautiful. It was much, much better than some of the gardens I had been to. When you get there, you can see just vast green lawns with rolling hills and shady trees in the background. It's also oozing with history as some of the generals during the Civil War were buried here.

It was in Kettering that I had my first experience in a local brewery, and I loved it. Aside from the fact that beers cost cheap per glass, I got to sit down and talk to some of the locals. It's a crazy, but very laid-back way to hang out. I also got to watch a nice music festival in Franze Pavilion. According to locals, some concerts of celebrities here can cost as little as $5. How nice is that?

# Part 9

# A Grueling but Rewarding Job in Pennsylvania

One of my avid interests aside from science and traveling is history. Although I enjoy natural landscapes like hiking trails, lakes, gardens, and parks, I am more enamored with old structures and stories about the destination. Perhaps it has something to do with my penchant for recollecting my short life in Jamaica. Moreover, history tells a lot not only about the place but also about its people.

So, when I was offered by the agency to work in Pennsylvania, I just had to grab the chance. I longed to see the birthplace of this country's independence.

The state shares a border with Ohio, New Jersey, Delaware, West Virginia, and at some points Ontario in Canada. It has a total land area of roughly 47,000 square miles, making it one of the top 35 states in the country with a total population of more than 12 million. It has one of the highest population densities in the United States.

Like a huge part of the United States, the state used to be a home for so many Native American nations such as, the Iroquois, Shawnee, and Delaware. However, as Europeans came around and established their place in America, they were driven off. Some of them traveled to other states and assimilated with the rest of the population. The first settlers were the Swedish and the Dutch that wished to make it the New Netherland. However, the state eventually became the land of the Quaker because of William Penn, from whose name Pennsylvania was based from. Soon more Quakers and Europeans arrived, dominating the state in the middle of the eighteenth century.

Pennsylvania produced one president, James Buchanan, and was one of the first states to ratify the country's Constitution. The city of Philadelphia became the convening venue for the Founding Fathers. The vote of a Pennsylvanian, John Morton, was believed to have sealed the deed and granted everyone's independence. Simply put, the state played a very huge role in the declaration of independence and the creation of the U.S. Constitution. The official nickname of the state, Keystone State, is also related to this momentous event in history.

## What Am I Doing Here?

As a traveling histologist, I get to work with different types of jobs in various health care facilities. When I was in Pennsylvania, I was assigned in one of the most advanced health care systems that I had ever been.

I could not articulate properly how overwhelmed I was with all the technologies and knowledge overflowing here. I was surely nervous, since I was not exposed to all of these high-tech devices before, but I was very glad to have found expert guidance from the seniors and my other colleagues. It helped too that I worked on day shifts. I can rest properly at night or take some time to roam around Pittsburgh, where I worked.

This health care facility was not just about taking care of patients, but they are also trying to make breakthroughs. That is the part that truly thrilled me the most. I know that I will never be recognized as part of whatever gets to be discovered here, but being able to contribute was more than enough for me.

During weekends, I usually left my apartment to see what Pittsburgh has to offer. Of course, I started with cultural and historical sites such as the Senator John Heinz Pittsburgh History Center located downtown and within the Strip District, which is the go-to place for entertainment, dining, and shopping. This center contains galleries occupying more than five levels, all of them telling you of the very long history of the state, starting from over 200 years ago. If you are into the arts, you should never miss the museum dedicated to Andy Warhol. I love to go there on Fridays since I get to experience more than just the paintings; the museum becomes more alive with music and other types of performances. The legacy of the Carnegies are also found everywhere in Pittsburgh, including in a center for natural history.

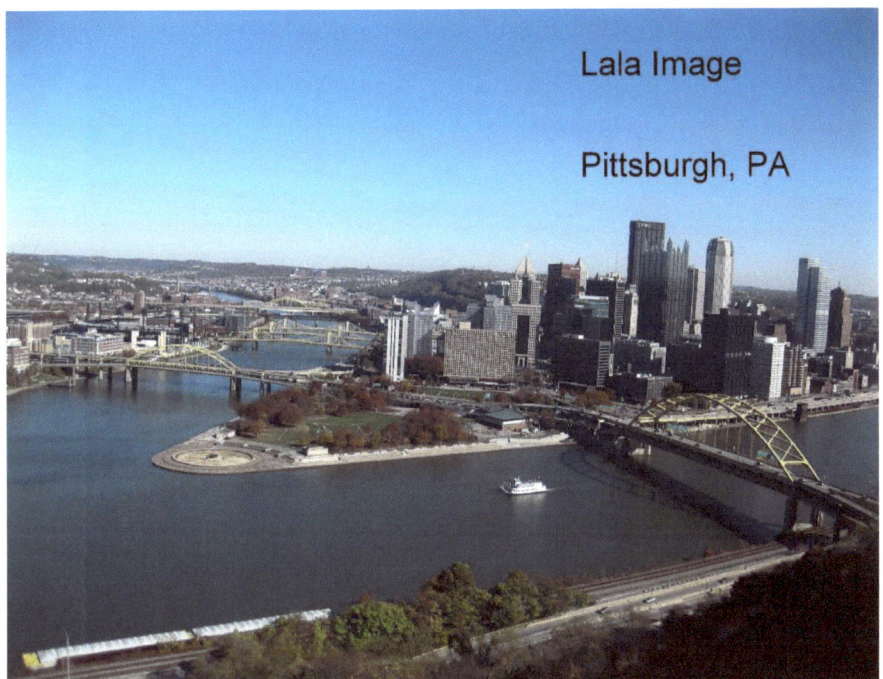

One of the favorite tourist destinations is the Phipps Conservatory and Botanical Garden of Henry Phipps, who accumulated vast wealth through his steel business. It is 19th-century garden and conservatory that is deeply inspired by the glass houses during the Victorian Era. Even if you are not such a big fan of plants, you will surely appreciate the simplicity but beauty of your surroundings.

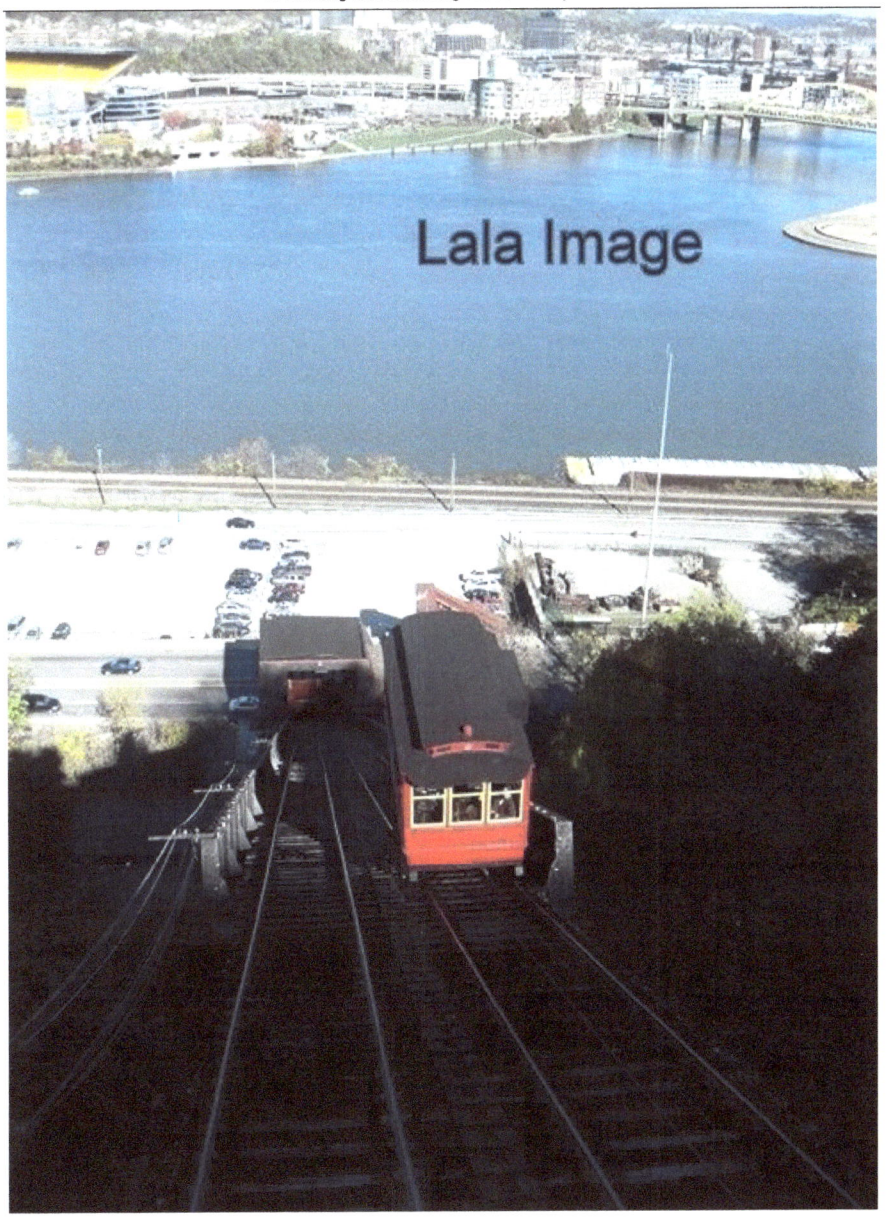

In the middle of the city is one of the biggest fountains in the whole wide world. It marks your presence in the Point State Park, which was created to honor the British. If you are not afraid of heights, you may want to experience a very steep incline ride toward the top. Called the Duquesne Incline, it is located on West Carson Street. It was built sometime in the 1870s, but it was restored almost a century after. Much of what it looked like in the original had been preserved, so being inside was already a tour back in time.

One day off from work, a good friend brought me to the University of Pittsburgh, which was a very gorgeous and large school. He then took me to Cathedral of Learning and into the Nationality Rooms. Now if you are wondering why it is called as such, well, it is because each room was a tribute to every ethnicity that made the city what it is now. For me, that is such a cool way to display and remember history. There are more than 20 of these rooms and these include Indian, Polish, African, Chinese, French, Welsh, and Italian.

The farthest I had gone to was Lancaster County to see a real Amish village. The Amish cannot really interact with us, but the guide was very helpful in answering our questions. Seeing how they thrived with utmost simplicity was remarkable. It made me realize that a person can live without some conveniences if he wills it.

# Part 10

# The World of Surgery in North Carolina

I have to say it took me a while to get acclimated with North Carolina. Although I spent a part of my childhood in Jamaica, I was actually a city girl through and through having fully immersed myself into the culture and lifestyle in New York.

I am not saying that North Carolina is not urban, but most of the best attractions are actually its nature. Though, I guess that is the great thing about traveling: it opens you to a whole new world. If you can be more receptive to the brand-new opportunities, you will discover how truly beautiful a place is. It is definitely what I experienced when I stayed here.

In North Carolina, I was assigned in the general hospital with a surgical department. I was responsible for taking care and handling the specimens properly. I was dealing with both normal and abnormal tissues, particularly, if they are cancer related.

My work demanded that I report at night, but once you are in there, you can never truly feel the eeriness or the loneliness of the night since people just came and went out of the hospital doors! The lab almost never ran out of things to do, which was definitely good for me since I did not have the chance to notice the time.

I was lucky to find an apartment quite close to the facility, so I did not have to travel for some time; rest was quite easy for me. Nevertheless, I developed a ritual of dropping off at the local café down by the corner where I lived to have a nice cup of freshly brewed coffee or, if I felt ravenous, a heavy breakfast of two layers of pancakes with organic honey. The scent of their meals was simply incredible, and it never failed to make me feel quite happy. It had been a great pick-me-up and perhaps an awesome way to start a brand-new day.

## What Is Up, North Carolina?

One of the things I liked most about North Carolina was that it is very close to Virginia, where I attended college. North Carolina is located in the South and shares borders with Tennessee, Georgia, and, of course, South Carolina. Its landscape is very varied with mountains situated hundreds of feet above sea level, yet it actually faces the Atlantic Ocean, which is found in its east. When it comes to land area, it is only 28th, but it belongs to the top 10 most populous states in the country.

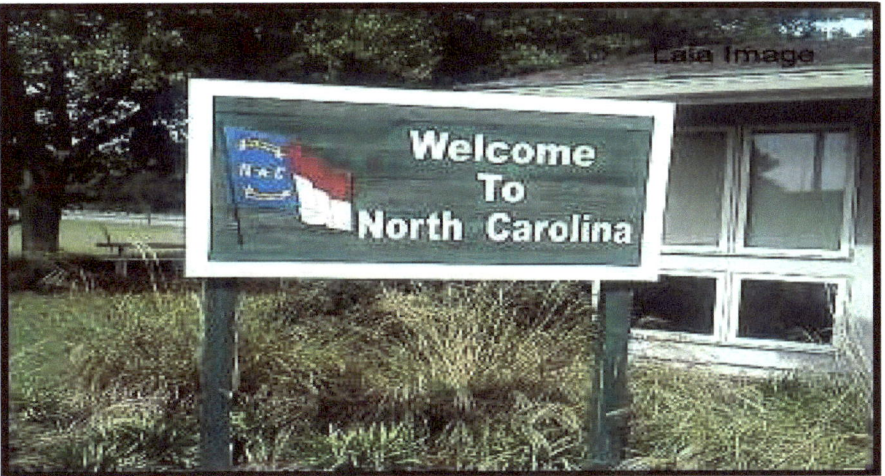

The climate of NC can also be very different, depending on where you are. If you are located in the plains, you will find the summers to be more humid with less rain. Winters are also usually mild. When you are in the region of Piedmont, weather can become a bit more extreme.

NC for me is highly ideal for the adventurous. Although I am more of "gallery and museum" girl, I was lucky to have found friends who encouraged me to try out something new. One of the first places I visited when I was in NC was the Grandfather Mountain. We spent around 2 days here, and even then I felt those were not enough! The mountain, which is more than 4,000 feet above the sea, was simply breathtaking. You know, I have been to a couple of hikes before, and they normally started out exciting until such feeling tapered because you hardly see anything worth interesting. Well, it is different when you are here.

I walked across the hanging bridge, which gave me a majestic view of the mountains and the natural habitats of bears, eagles, and river otters, to name a few. Unlike commercial zoos, they roamed around their natural habitats with ideal enclosure, so you can observe them as close as you can without sacrificing your own safety.

By the next week, they took me to Great Smoky Mountains as well as to Pigsah National Forest the week after.

I spent most of my time in Charlotte, however, since this is where the facility is located. I got to fully enjoy my time in museums such as Carolinas Aviation Museum, Mint Museum, and Levine Museum.

On Fridays, my colleagues and I normally enjoyed some night life like in Big Ben Pub and Restaurant in South Boulevard. We also had a great time in Carolina Ale House and All American Pub. When it comes to barbecue, I would highly recommend BarBQ King in Wilkinson Boulevard and Buffalo Wild Wings. If you truly want to eat a lot, then you can go for a Food Tour, which include a visit in the local breweries, wine classes, and of course lots of eating and cooking.

Charlotte has a lot of beautiful paved paths that you would not mind simply walking. Once, I came across a tour group that enjoyed the city by a Segway. I had not ridden a Segway since it looked quite dangerous for me, but it seemed the riders had a fantastic time. On the other hand, if you would not like the Segway, then go rent a bike! If I had my way, I would have bought or rented a bike so that I can see the entire city!

Ah, North Carolina is sparkling with new things for me. I am so happy that I was able to embrace it after a while because I learnt to take full advantage of what it offers. It is just too bad when I was having a fun time, I had to leave and move onto my next destination.

# Part 11

# Quite a Tough Time
# in Washington State

Every time I tried to describe my job to friends and family, they often can't help but feel envious. I must admit that I am indeed very lucky. Not everyone is given the chance to do the things they love, much less travel and be provided with a lot of benefits.

On the other hand traveling can also be very lonely. It is like literally living in a suitcase. There were many times when I missed my family back home and real home-cooked meals from Mom. There came a point when I did not want to be too attached with the people I met and worked with since I will be leaving anyway. I can get too attached to a place and find it truly hard to say goodbye. Sometimes it felt that I was always starting from scratch.

Then there is of course the state's climate, which can become very terrible. Overcast skies and gloomy weather seemed to have a huge effect on me as they can easily dampen my spirit.

When I moved to Washington State, after my contract in North Carolina ended, it was in the middle of January, when the temperature was definitely low and the surroundings were very cold. Moreover, because of the topography and location of the state, rains were very common, and sometimes road got flooded.

Perhaps to make things worse was the fact that I worked not in the best health care facility. It was definitely not a Seattle Grace Hospital! I was normally left to my own devices, perhaps because they believed I had already gained considerable experience in my field. My depression was an all time high, and for some reason, more people were diagnosed with multiple sclerosis.

Multiple Sclerosis (MS) comes in varying degrees, but usually it is a gradual disintegration of the body and its function, so I know how very hard it is to have one. There was also a rapid onset of breast cancer cases.

Although we were making progress in breast cancer, it still remains one of the number one killers among different types of cancer. Further, people have the misconception that only women develop it. No! Even men do; in fact, it is more dangerous in men because of such misconception. Since they think they could not get it, they often ignore lumps or do not perform breast checks themselves.

With so many serious diseases brought to the hospital, it did not come as a surprise that our workload was heavy for most nights. Hence, during weekends, I always made sure that I can unwind.


## Washington Comforted Me

Stress may be overwhelming, not to mention the occasional feelings of loneliness and aloneness, but fortunately Washington State was there to cheer me up. It has a great balance between urbanity and nature, and the people were truly friendly and accommodating. It has an excellent standard of living too. You are paid well, but the costs of commodities are not very high. While writing this chapter, I came across an article that said *Forbes* has just considered the state as the best to earn a living — I can surely vouch for that.

Washington is a very large state; it is among the top 20 states in the country based in land size. It has a total area of more than 70,000 square miles. Its capital is Olympia, but its most popular city is Seattle. More than 55% of its total population lives here! Obviously, the state was named after the first president of the United States, George Washington.

The state is nicknamed Evergreen State because it is abundant with evergreens. This may explain too why lumber still remains a well-known job or industry in Washington.

Many people tend to confuse Washington State with Washington DC. They are definitely different from each other. While Washington is a recognized state, DC (or District of Columbia) is a district and is the appointed capital of the country. Almost everyone who lives here have jobs in various areas of the government and international organizations. I can talk more about DC in the later pages since I got a chance to visit it.

I spent most of my time in Seattle since it was where I lived when I was in Washington. To be honest, I was happy to be here since I secretly admired the city especially when I got to watch *Sleepless in Seattle* when I was still young. Definitely, as homage to the movie, one of my first tourist destinations was the Space Needle. You can never miss it, as it is a long-standing symbol of the vibrant city. One of the tallest landmarks or structures in the United States, it is meant to be an observation deck. It was built during the World's Fair in 1962. It gives tourists 360-degree view of the city and the nearby mountains and other landscapes, as well as other regions. It also has its own restaurant and function rooms for private events.

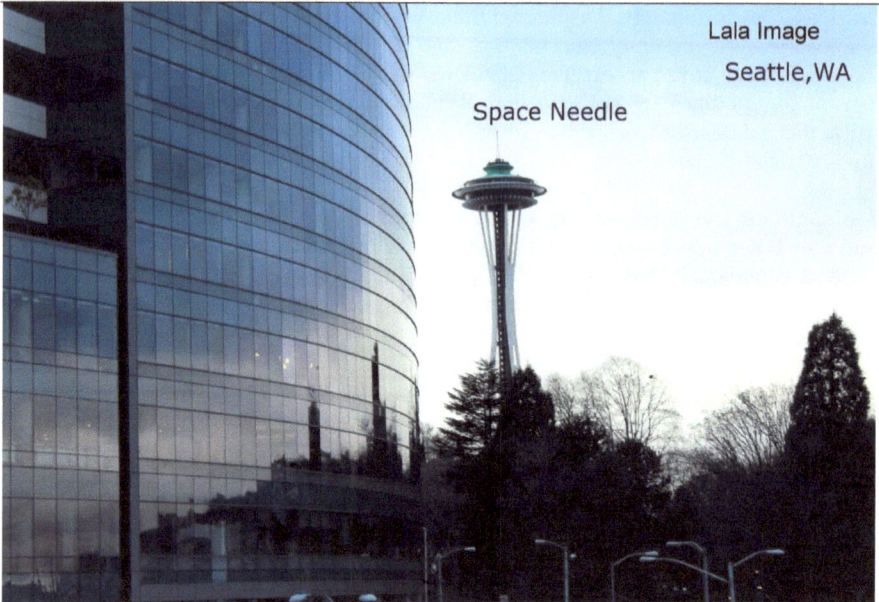

On Sundays, I would head to Pike Place for fresh produce and eat! I also visited the Museum of Flight and Woodland Park Zoo.

My trip to Vancouver (not to be confused with Vancouver of Canada) was filled with lots of history. I checked out Pearson Air Museum and Clark County Historical Museum. Since I arrived on a weekend, by Sunday my friends and I heard mass in Proto-Cathedral of St. James the Greater, which was built sometime in the 19th century. Then we went to Vancouver Lake Park for some sightseeing. In Vancouver, you can find the home of Ulysses Grant, the U.S.'s former president and an influential commander during the Civil War.

My journey in Washington wasn't all rosy, but it was humbling. I think I've never helped as many people as I did when I was here. That made my job more gratifying. Most of all, I became to understand why, despite the crazy climate, many loved Washington so much.

# Part 12

# Leisurely Trips to Missouri and Washington DC

Although I usually travel for work, there are times when I go to certain places with no career agenda. I did that in four incredible states.

## Hello, Missouri!

When I was still working in Indiana, I had some colleagues and friends who came from Missouri, and they had nothing but good things to say about the place. Since there was enough gap between my next contract after Indiana, I took the time to visit the state.

Missouri is 21st in terms of land area, measuring almost 70,000 miles. It has a total population of 6 million, making it among the top 20 most populous states in the country.

It is also referred to as the Show Me State, which I found out, has a very interesting back story, depending on who is talking to you. One attributed it to the Missouri miners working in Colorado. They required frequent repetitions of directions, so it became a sort of joke among the miners and pit bosses — since they were from Missouri and they did not immediately understand instructions, they needed demos all the time.

The most popular one was in reference to William Duncan Vandiver who served as the state's congressman many years ago. In one of his speeches, he claimed that since he was from Missouri, he would not be persuaded by glowing speeches but by proof and example. In other words, people of Missouri were highly skeptical and stubborn.

The truth is, I did not see any of these characteristics when I went to visit the state, though I would say that they were excellent conversationalists.

I stayed in Missouri for about a week, allowing me to see a good list of their popular attractions.

One of the first cities I visited was St. Louis. I am not a big fan of sports and their teams, but for me, seeing the people watching their favorite teams playing is a good way of knowing about their culture and behavior. So, one of the things I did was watched a game of St. Louis Cardinals. The stadium was literally jam-packed with people, and you can certainly feel their intensity toward the game. Of course, since I was there, I opted to cheer for the team too.

During nighttime, I headed to Westport Plaza, which was one of their bustling entertainment districts. A friend and I used to work together in Indiana and one of the reasons why I was in town — we headed for an awesome Japanese dinner in Drunken Fish. Their sushi is sensational! And I was very grateful for the people who taught me how to eat sushi properly so that I will not have to embarrass myself while dining. We then proceeded to Trainwreck Saloon for a couple of rounds of ladies' beer and beverages, simply having a fun and relaxing time. We stayed there until 11:00 p.m. After that, I went home to my hotel.

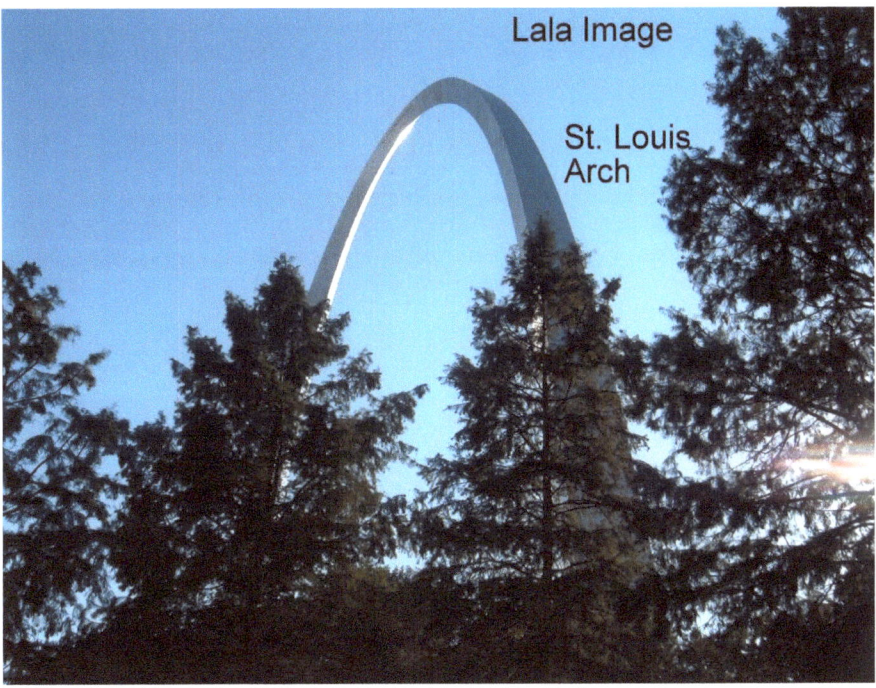

The next day, my friend along with her daughter and I took a road trip to Springfield. It was a good 3-hour drive along the I-44, and it was a good thing that there was no traffic. As soon as we arrived, we checked into our hotel and immediately began our sightseeing.

Since we had a kid in tow, one of the first places we went to was the Discovery Center, which was dear to us since we worked in the medical field or our job revolved around science. Well, most of our companions were children since I think it was truly built for them, but it did not really matter to us adults. We always believed that we were kids at heart! The unassuming building offers different levels of exhibits including a section about dinosaurs and explorations. Almost all their exhibits are interactive, so the kids are allowed to dig into soil and look for fossils like dinosaur bones. We then went to Jordan Valley Ice Park to see a hockey game before we went out for late lunch in a barbecue restaurant.

Back in our hotel, I did more research about cool attractions nearby, and I chanced upon Gillioz Theater, which was actually a restored 1920s theater. Fortunately, there was a play scheduled on the day, and it was kid-friendly. I thought it was a great way to cap our first day in Springfield.

The next day we traveled for around 30 minutes through W Melville Road and arrived at Fantastic Caverns in N. Farm Road. You will never really miss it since it had this huge signboard located outside.

Since it was still 30 minutes before their opening hour, I was really thinking we were quite early for our ride to the cavern, but I was pleasantly surprised when a long line was already waiting for us. Anyway, we were part of the second batch.

The trip inside was nothing short of amazing, and the experience was captivating. It was truly an underground cave! While in most caves you had to make your own trek, which can sometimes be dangerous, here everyone had to ride a tram drawn by a jeep. Thus, it remained comfortable for all of us, and quite odd, our path was like paved because the ride was very smooth all throughout.

While riding, the guide will be there to talk more about the cave, such as its history and the interesting things you will see along the way such as the Saw Tooth, Soda Straws, Salamander, and the amazing Hall of Giants whose sheer size can definitely overwhelm you and yet leave you in awe.

We stayed in the area for about 2 hours and even bought our souvenirs from the gift shop. After that, we went back to our hotel to take our lunch before we left for St. Louis.

From St. Louis, I traveled alone to Jefferson City and stayed there for 3 days, visiting their eerie State Penitentiary, taking a guided tour to the Governor's Mansion where the present governor lives, and the Cole County Historical Museum, which houses many artworks from Europe such as France.

## Goodness, Washington DC

If I were given a chance, I would probably spend an entire year in Washington DC. Now that may sound too much for a tourist to do, and note everyone likes DC, but can you ever complain when I just love museums? This place has one of the biggest concentrations of museums that it will take me at least a week to visit all of them, and I cannot even explore each one of them fully then.

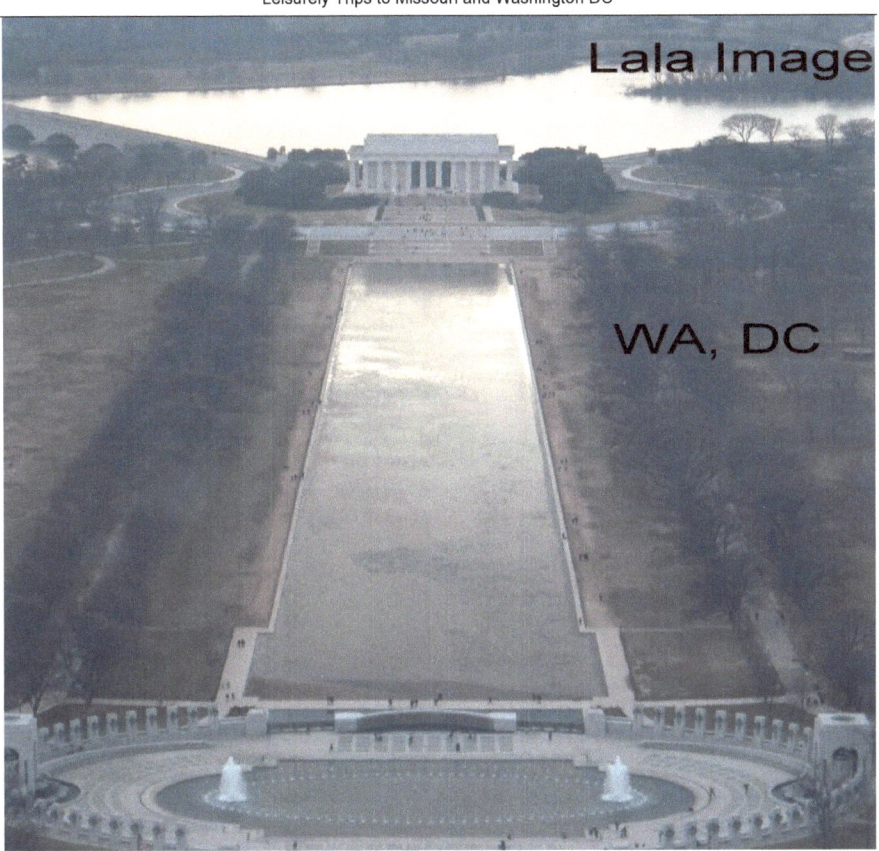

Many people tend to confuse Washington State with DC simply because they share a name, but as I mentioned in the previous chapter, DC is a federal district, not a state. It was created by 1700s since the leadership at the time thought the country needed to have a capital that is not within a state. It was formed on a land which its nearest states, Virginia, and Maryland, donated a portion of their land. It is actually a small piece of land, covering less than 200 square kilometers, and more than 600,000 people live here. However, it is easy for the population to swell because of the tourists and commuters who live in the nearby states. Its size earned it the American Rome, perhaps in reference to Vatican, which is one of the smallest countries in the world, the seat of Roman Catholicism, and a country found within a country that is Italy. It is also referred to as DC, Nation's Capital, Capital City, and at some point Nation's Capital sometime in the 1990s because of its very high crime rate (which is kind of ironic since the seat of government is here; police visibility and protection should be very high).

61

I visited Washington DC quite a few times when I was still in Virginia, but I never had the opportunity to fully explore it. So when I had enough time to go back home before my next assignment, I opted to schedule a 5-day tour to the district. Since it is just a small place with a lot of structures and people, traffic can be a huge problem. So, what I would normally do is to ride the Virginia Railway Express.

As I talked earlier, DC has many museums — and I truly mean many. Imagine, in a small tract of land, there are more than 50 of them! The great thing is that most of them are free or, if not, a lot cheaper than other museums in the country. So traveling on a budget here is definitely not a problem at all.

The first order of the day is visiting the Smithsonian. It is an institution that is purposely set up by Congress, which explains its location and significance. There are many museums under the Smithsonian, such as Museum of American History, Museum of the American Indian, and Museum of Natural History. The highlight, however, will be the Smithsonian Institution Building, which is also commonly referred to as the Castle. It is a 19th-century building that now serves as the main information center and where the administrative offices can be found. The building, nevertheless, is a gem since it also has some wonderful exhibits like Schermer Hall and Smithson Crypt. My day tour included a look at the grand Washington Monument, Declaration of Independence Memorial, and Lincoln Memorial and its reflecting pool.

Of course, a trip to Washington DC will never be complete without seeing the National Mall, and I did that at night since it looked incredibly amazing around this time than in the morning, and I did not have to fight for its view with other tourists.

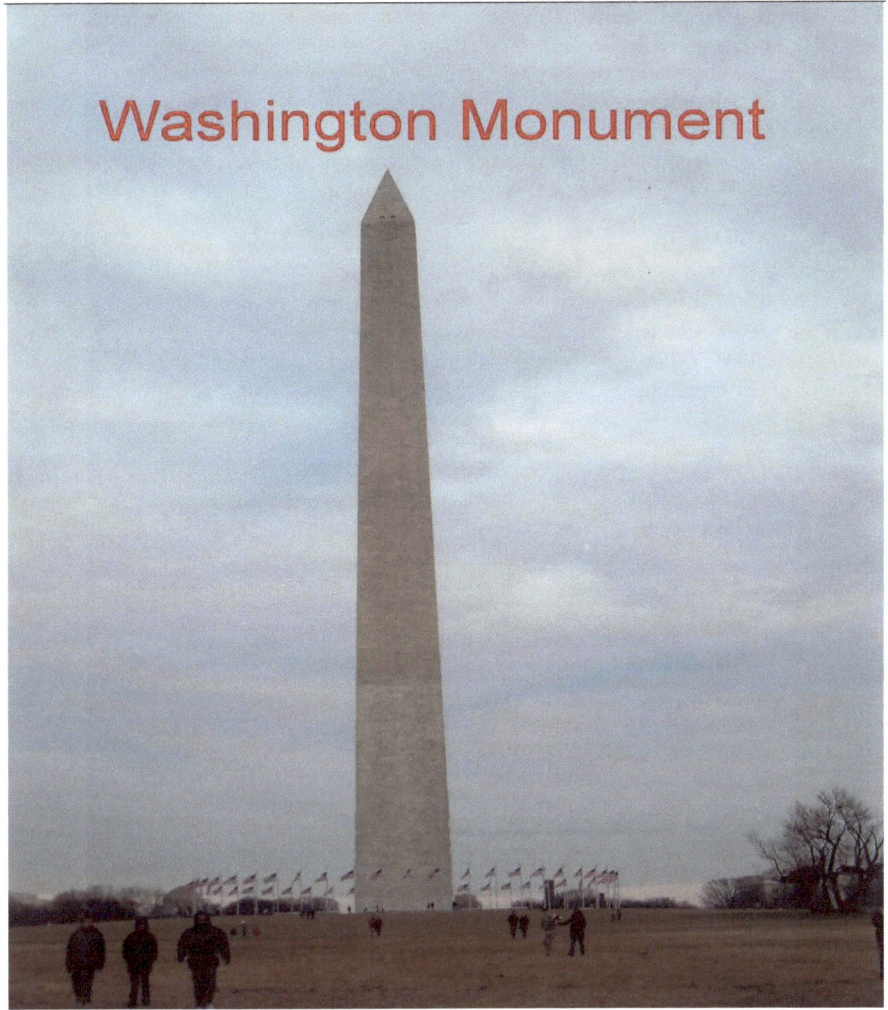

Riding a Metrorail and armed with my only luggage, a backpack, I went from Downtown to south portion of DC, in Georgetown. It was not as crowded as downtown and offers few attractions, but I liked my time there since it was stress free. Moreover, it has a very laid-back yet affluent approach, and walking around it made me think that maybe I was in Europe!

The Dumbarton Oaks is one of the most visited places in Georgetown, and that is definitely understandable. Aside from its huge role in the country's independence — it was where the charter for the United Nations was drawn — it is made even lovelier because of its sprawling, well-manicured gardens that will surely remind you of the Victorian Era. In fact, I was so close to donning on a costume. It was just perfect. There is a garden for herbaceous plants, vegetable garden, and cut-flower garden. If you want to see the best parts of the garden, it is best if you can take the guided tour, which I did.

I then rented a bike that took me to Georgetown University. As expected not all of it is accessible, but I was not really interested much on its buildings rather on the Exorcist Steps. If you are wondering why it is called such, it is because it was featured in the horror movie! It is where Father Damian Karras met his untimely end. It is a very narrow set of steps that is so popular. You should not be surprised if you see people trying to pretend they have died after falling off the stairs—yup, a fitting tribute to the movie.

I stayed for another day in Georgetown seeing Old Stone House, Tudor Place, House of Sweden, and the two well-known cemeteries, Oak Hill and Mount Zion.

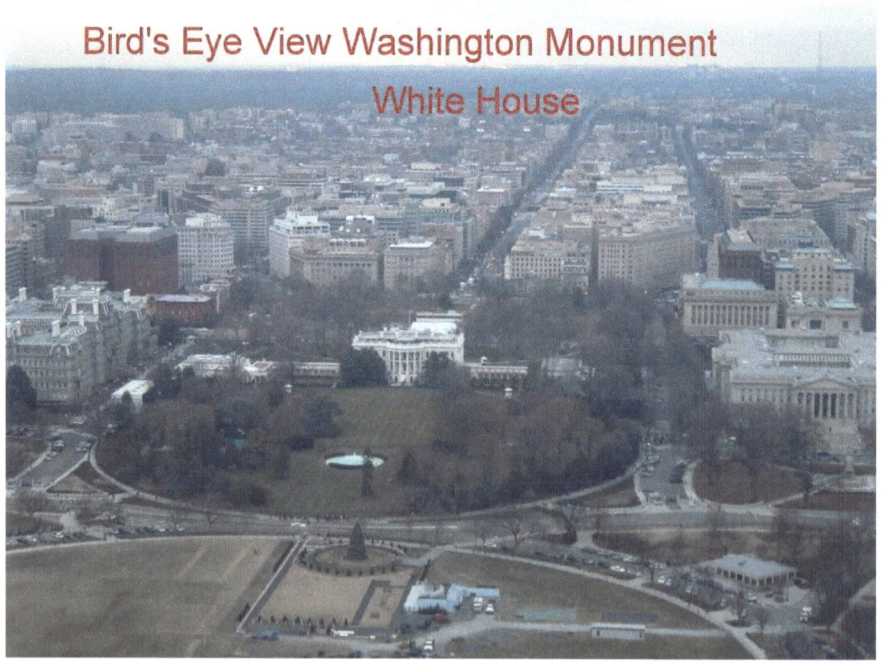

Bird's Eye View Washington Monument
White House

Many people think that Washington DC is expensive. Well, I think every place is if you don't set a budget. I always do. To help you save money, start with the free tours and attractions first. Downtown alone has Friendship Park, lobby of Willard Intercontinental, Arlington National Cemetery, Gravelly Point, and the fresh market in Dupont Circle. Many museums are free on certain days as well. Since, public transport is the way to go in here, you'll save more money.

# Part 13

# New York, New York

*Alicia Keys could have never been correct when she sang, "in New York, concrete jungle where dreams are made of. There's nothing you can't do!" Whenever I hear that line, I can never forget my experience in one of the best cities in the world.*

*As mentioned in my previous chapters, right after I graduated pre-med in Virginia, I took a job that allowed me to go back to New York – the first state where I stayed after we moved from Jamaica. Although I moved from one facility to another, there's only one thing that ties them all together: they are some of the best in the country and perhaps the entire world. The job may have been more grueling since we're serving hundreds of patients, but I can never discount the fact that I learnt so much in NY.*

*New York is understandably demanding; considering that most of the hospitals there also accept patients from all around the globe. Since we are needed almost nonstop, we took different shifts to ensure there's always someone who can process the tissues and other specimens.*

*Nevertheless, it has proven to be one huge playground that it no longer mattered if I left the hospital in the dead of winter or in the unholy hours before the break of dawn – there's always a place to go to, a new experience to take in.*

## A Short Background about New York

New York is perhaps one of the most popular states in the country owing to the fact that it's a melting pot for those who want to live their American dream. If you don't know it yet, Ellis Island was formerly an immigration center. Throngs of Europeans who wanted to escape the war or dazzled by the magnificent stories about America were brought there and processed. Those who passed the immigration were then taken to the main island. Since many of them didn't have a lot of money for travel and accommodation, most settled in New York.

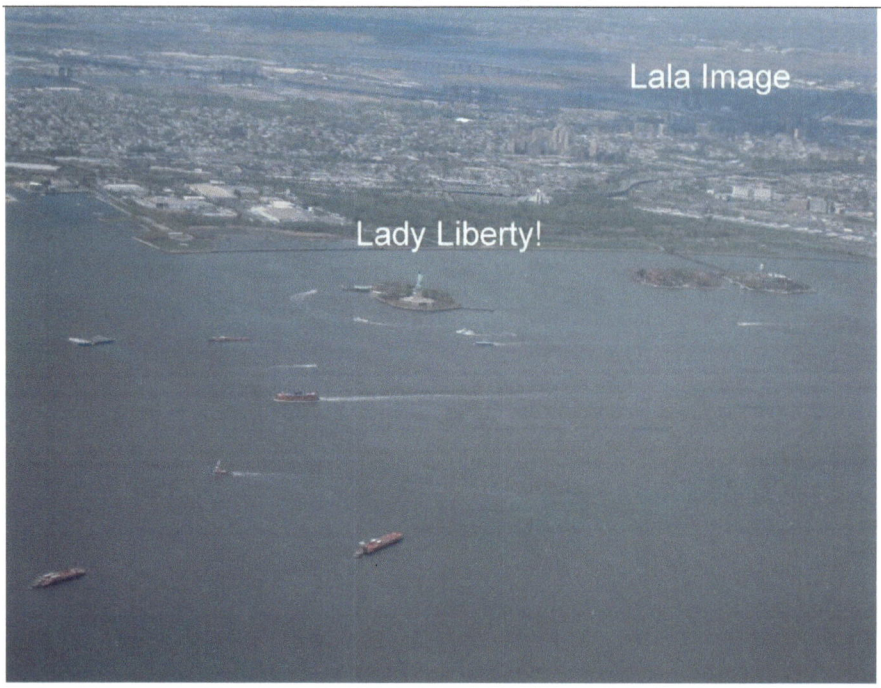

New York is one of the smallest states at no more than 55,000 square miles, but it's one of the most populous states with over 19 million residents. That basically explains why the cost of living here, especially the accommodation or home, is higher than other states, even when compared to its neighbors such as New Jersey. It's pretty normal for people in here to share an apartment or live in a very tight space. Over 35 percent of NY residents, however, are right in New York City, which includes the Bronx, Brooklyn, Manhattan, Staten Island, and Queens.

New York has a lot of nicknames, which I think is just very common among U.S. states, but the one that is the most popular is the Empire State. It may have something to do with the Empire State Building, which remains one of the tallest structures in the country. Back then, it was a symbol of the city's wealth and economic prominence. It seems like even today it has retained such status.

## What to See

You will never run out of things to see and do in New York. For example, if you're looking for "free," all you have to do is go to Central Park, which is actually a very huge tract of land that covers more than 700 acres right in the heart of the city. Sometimes, when I am really tired, I would just be right here, sitting in one of its benches, observing people jogging, walking, having a picnic, or playing. I feel reenergized by the serenity and beauty of the park.

There are many things to do in Central Park too aside from people watching. Right inside the park is a zoo as well as a conservatory garden, which features plants that came all the way from Europe. The garden, which is divided into different sections, is also inspired by the grand manicured lawns and gardens of the Europeans, like those in Italy and France. You can also climb a castle or walk on quaint bridges. Of course, food will never be out of sight.

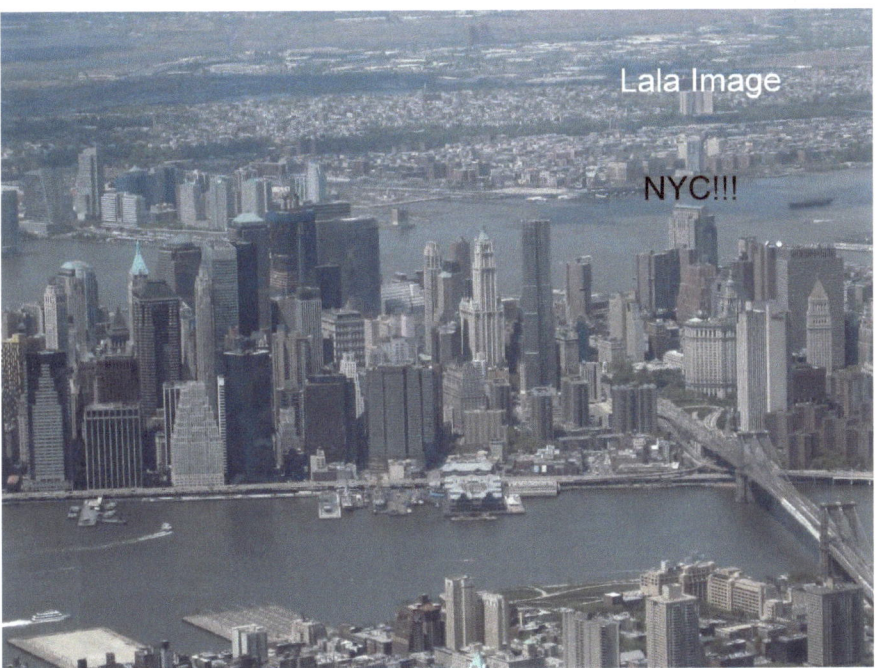

Aside from Central Park, there's also the ever-famous Statue of Liberty, which was a gift from France to the United States as a way of forging their friendship. It is located in Liberty Island, which is completely uninhabited. To get there, therefore, you need to ride a boat. Being one of the most well-known attractions in New York, you better make sure that you can reserve your tickets beforehand. There are special reservations if you want to climb all the way to its crown and pedestal.

During Christmas, whenever I am in New York, I try my best to drop by the

Rockefeller Center. The Christmas spirit is very much alive here since it's where you can find the giant Christmas tree and the popular ice skating rink. Definitely, included in the itinerary is a memorable trip to Macy's for their beautiful Christmas decors.

You also must not miss out Times Square, especially if you're into broadways or musicals. In fact, you don't need to be avid fans of these. Just being there gives you a different vibe that makes New York also an excellent center of culture and the arts. Speaking of arts, I highly suggest that you also explore the Metropolitan Museum of Art, American Museum of Natural History, and Museum of Modern Art.

## Manhattan's Skyline

The skyline of Manhattan has been featured many times in movies, music videos, magazines, and other materials; but still it's a totally different feeling when you're up there. The word "magic" seems like an understatement. Being up there, I thought about how small I was compared to the majesty of New York, and yet there I was, making my dream come true and standing proud and tall because of what I have achieved so far.

One of the best ways to see the skyline is through the Empire State Building. This still remains to be a commercial center, and there are very huge businesses operating in here. Yet it also understands its value in U.S. history. Thus, it allows locals and tourists alike to experience its grandness. There are two floors where you can see the Manhattan skyline from the Empire State. You can go to the 86th floor, which requires a ticket, but it gives you a 360-degree view. There's a smaller one that is open to the public right at 102nd floor. If you get too dizzy because of the height, you can choose the Skyride on the second floor, which is basically a motion simulator of the city; it lasts for about 25 minutes. Another way to experience the skyline is by checking out restaurants that are found several floors high. The views may not be as comparable as those in the Empire State, but they may appear to be much cheaper, and you don't need to fight your space with hundreds of other tourists or visitors.

## Upstate New York

Most of the tourists or visitors get to experience only a small portion of the state. This is because they forget that Upstate New York is incredibly beautiful too. In fact, if one wants to get away from the busy city life, all they need to do is go upstate!

For example, Hudson Valley offers some of the best-tasting wines in the country, not to mention a nice cruise along the Hudson River. The Finger Lakes, which got its name from the way it looks from an aerial satellite, has a lot of museums and of course lakes that you can explore. Most of the NY vineyards are also found in here.

Central New York, meanwhile, is famous for its great schools such as Syracuse University and Cornell University.

# Part 14

# Sunny California

Nothing can be as diverse as California when it comes to people. If you want to be educated about different cultures, well, this is where you should be. It has a very interesting mix of other large ethnic groups, including Latin Americans or Hispanic — specifically within a portion of Mexico called Baja, shares a border with California — Asians, and Native Americans. The state is also incredibly huge; you will surely have a lot of things to look forward to here.

In order for me not to feel burnt out with being a traveling histologist, I make it a point to visit other places mainly for pleasure. I decided to choose California because, aside from the fact that I hadn't been there before, it's a very popular state with many stories that captured its beauty, charm, and even notoriety.

Although California may sound very big because of its equally large and vibrant cities, it's not the largest state in the country; rather, more than 160,000 square miles, it ranks third. However, it's the most populous with more than 38 million people or roughly 250 people per square mile! That means that more than 12% of the entire people in the U.S. are right here. Can you imagine that? – but I guess that's what makes California even more special. A huge part of its character is derived from its culturally diverse people.

Since I only had a very limited time there, I wasn't able to see all California cities. Instead I picked Los Angeles, Pasadena, and San Francisco.

## City of Angels

When we talk about California, Los Angeles will always be hovering around that sometimes we forget that it's not the capital of the state rather Sacramento. Nevertheless, it's the biggest city in the state with almost 4 million people.

It took me a while to begin my tour in the city. I flew in, landed, and then got stuck in a very terrible traffic. It's a great thing that the driver had been conscious enough not to engage me in a conversation. I was dead tired from everything! After an hour, I arrived in my hotel, checked in, and slept for a few hours. When I was feeling refreshed, I then proceeded to my very first destination: the Getty Center.

If the name sounds familiar, well, because it is. Getty Center is the brainchild of J. Getty, built using a trust program. He's not only very rich, but he was also an avid collector of very valuable artworks, which he opted to share with the public than making more money out of them. In fact, he was so committed that his museum is actually free. You get to pay only when you have a car, yet fees are very cheap at $15 per car. It is reduced to $10 after 5:00 p.m. Since I just took a taxi, I didn't have to pay for anything.

Getty has a very impressive collection of art pieces, from old ones dating from the nineteenth century to the more contemporary artwork. So at some point, you can see the evolution of painting techniques and even subjects. The Central Garden is a sight to behold, which would have been more amazing if not for the smog in LA.

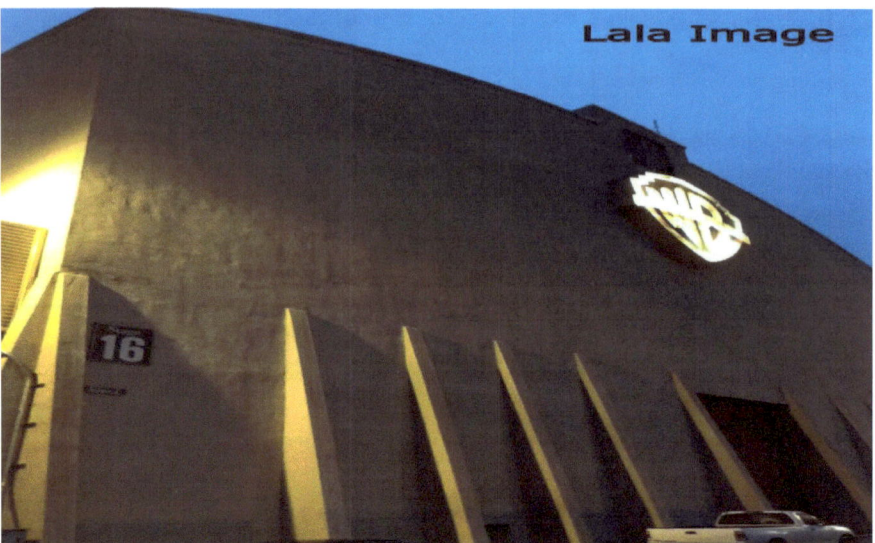

I grabbed a hefty dinner in the nearby café before I went to Rodeo Drive for some window-shopping. It's an elite strip of boutiques and dining places. I didn't have a lot of money with me, so I contented myself with looking at the window displays.

By the next day, I tried squeezing in a visit into space through the 80-year-old Griffith Observatory, Staples Center to watch the Lakers play (yes, I did it), and a self-guided tour around the famous Disney Concert Hall. A friend was also gracious enough to tour me around the Warner Brothers lot and on the iconic Hollywood Boulevard including, the Chinese Theater, Barnsdall Art Park, and the Hollywood Walk of Fame. In the evening, I had dinner at The Golden State to cap my very short tour in Los Angeles. By tomorrow, I'll be off to Pasadena.

Lala Image

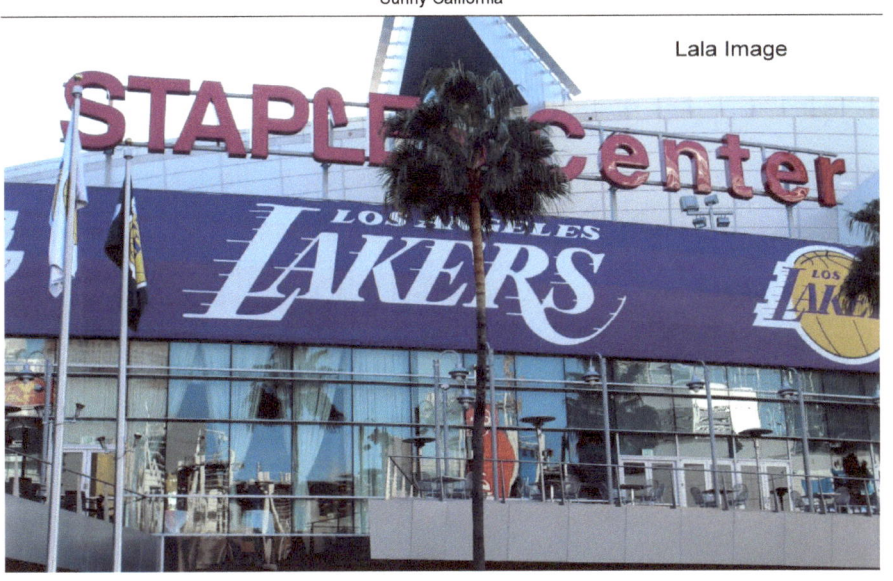

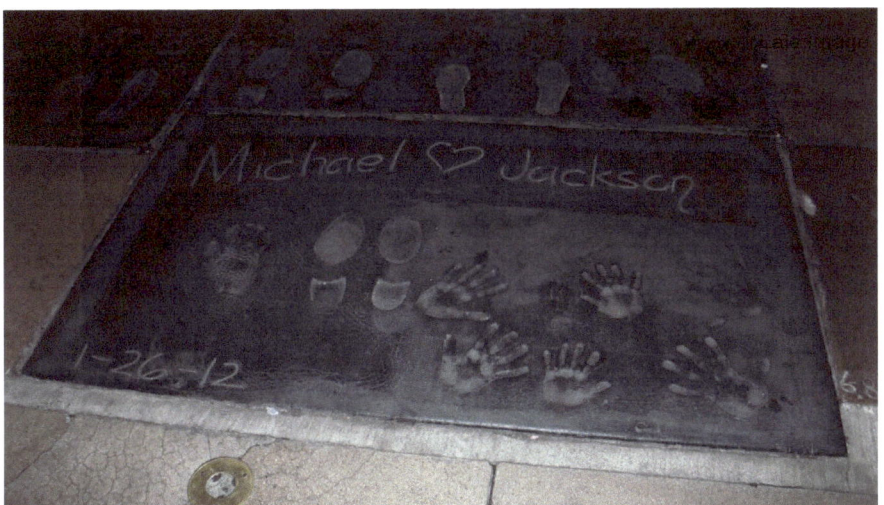

## Visual Arts in Pasadena

Since Pasadena is still part of the Los Angeles County, it isn't very far from Los Angeles City. In fact, it took me less than an hour to get there, including traffic.

Pasadena didn't have the same urban vibe as Los Angeles, but it's enriched by its culture, history, and arts. Its society of artists is considered as one of the regional centers for anything related to visual arts. It's also where you can find Bungalow Heaven, a very small close-knit community with homes built by craftsmen. Since it's already deemed a historical site, most of the houses had been restored and open to public on certain times of the year. Too bad I didn't make it to their annual home tour.

One of the highlights of my Pasadena visit was a tour around the Norton Simon Museum. Like the Getty Center, the pieces found here are private collections owned by Norton Simon. It took him more than 25 years to gather such a very impressive collection of artwork that includes paintings and sculptures. Some of his artworks are more than a century old, and many of his European paintings can be attributed to the Renaissance!

I also toured the Huntington Library for its gardens and Orange Grove Boulevard. Before I retired for the night, I also dropped by Old Pasadena.

## Why, Hello, San Francisco

From Pasadena, I traveled to Los Angeles airport and boarded a flight to San Francisco, which is almost like on the other side of California. Flight time was about an hour.

I once read a book where the gay character moved from his home state to San Francisco, because the latter was more accepting. You can say that it's always been ahead of the rest of the society's way of thinking. Compared to Los Angeles, I found SF to be more relaxed and casual

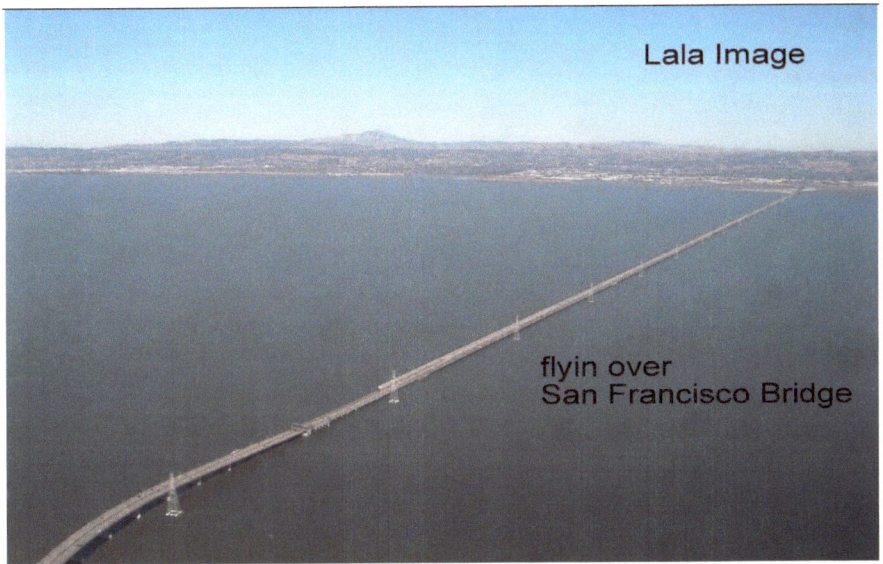

Lala Image

flyin over
San Francisco Bridge

I arrived quite early, so I had some enough time to freshen up and begin my tour with a ride in its world-famous cable car. It took me to some great neighborhoods that have populated the incline as well as districts like Chinatown, where I stopped. Chinatown here was certainly the largest I had ever been to that I ended up spending my entire morning here, checking out herbal shops, old banks like Bank of America, and their narrow alleys. I ended my tour with a nice bowl of steaming hot dim sum soup.

From Chinatown, I went to Walt Disney Museum, which was about 20 minutes away. It was a museum fit for the man who gave us Mickey Mouse and the rest of the Disney characters we've grown to love. Every gallery is a chronology of his life until his passing.

I stayed for only two days in San Francisco, but it was worth it. I rode a bike on the Golden Gate Bridge, checked out more exhibits in the Palace of Fine Arts, visited the Fisherman's Wharf and its nearby Ripley's, and shopped at Union Square.

Overall, California only rejuvenated my great love for arts, history, and culture, and I can't surely wait to go back when time permits.

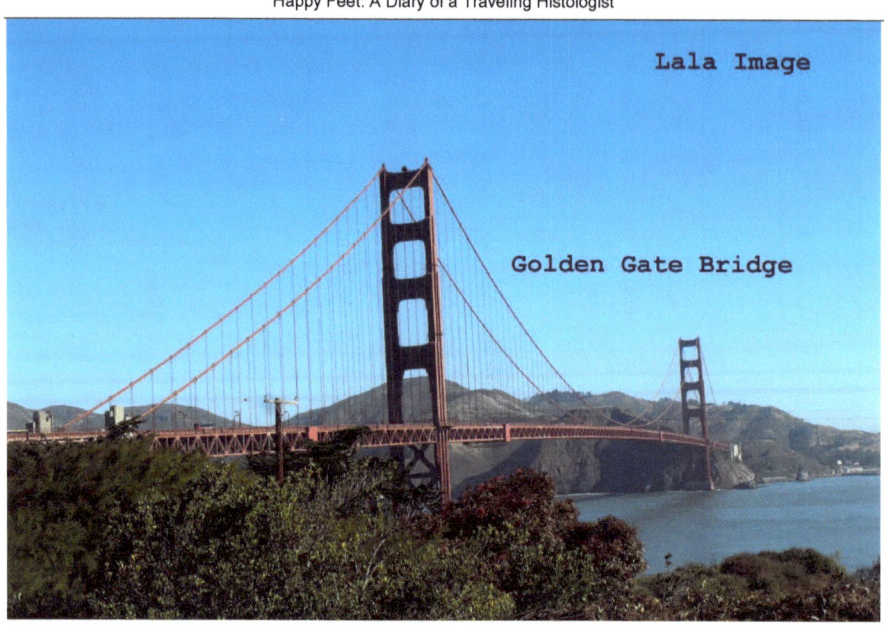

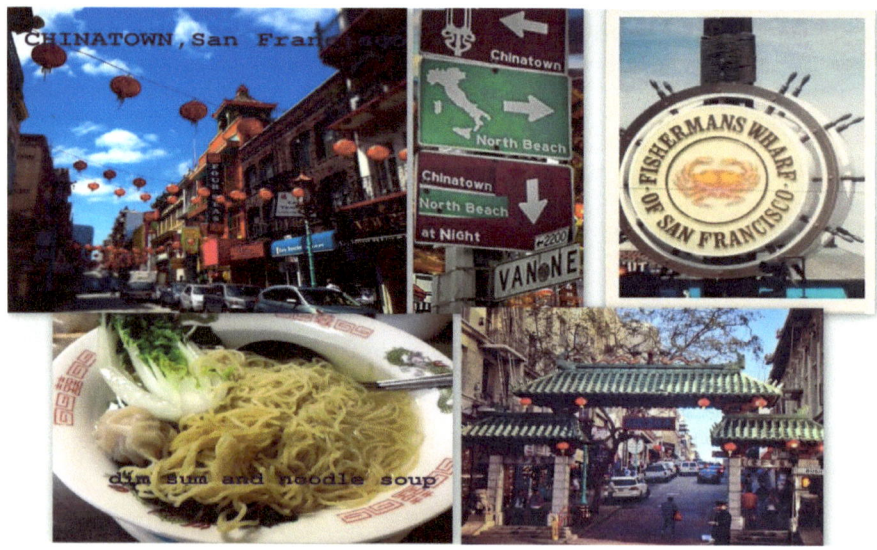

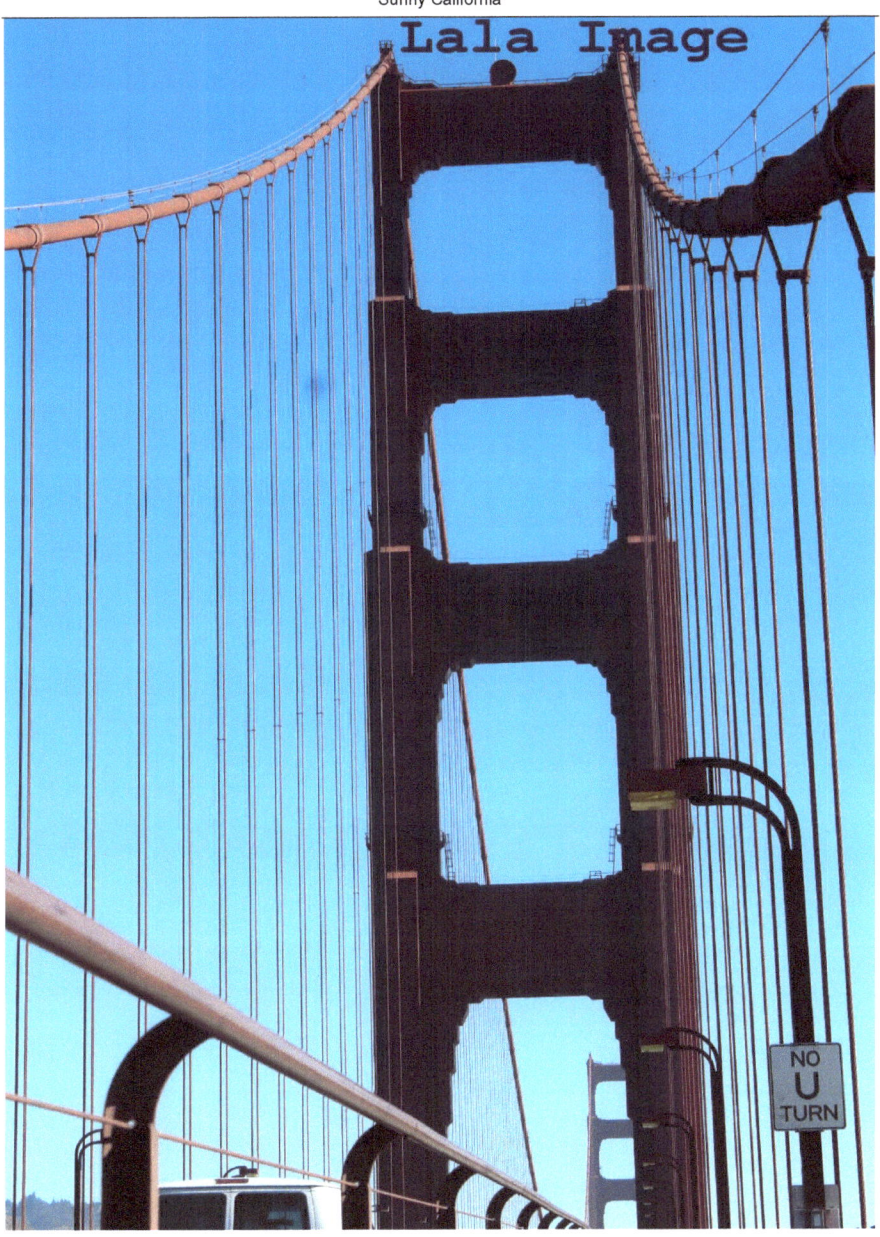

# Part 15

# Aloha, Hawaii

I have been around mainland USA traveling while doing my job, and so far, it has been a lot of fun. It felt like the entire country was my huge classroom where I learnt how to converse with different types of people, troubleshoot my own personal and professional issues, discover the beauty and eccentricity of every state, and appreciate their own culture, history, and heritage. I learnt to be less judgmental about others and realized that, in truth, America is not just for a certain group of people. It is for everyone who dared to dream and work as much as they can to reach it.

I wanted a bit of change — some twists in my scenery. Thus, after a few years of traveling within the mainland, I decided to fly to Hawaii.

Hawaii is incredibly different from the other states for a lot of reasons. First of all, it is the only state that is made up of islands and the other that is separated from the contiguous United States (the other being Alaska, the biggest state in terms of land area). Definitely, Virgin Islands is also an archipelago, but it is not really a state but a U.S. territory. Hawaii is located within the Pacific Ocean and is considered more of a Polynesian Island.

Second, it took a while before Hawaii became an official U.S. state. While most of the states in mainland United States were already declared as part of the country as early as the 1800s, this one was counted only during the 1950s. It is the last state to be included, so to speak.

Third, the state is mostly populated by Asians, which make up more than 38% of the population by 2010. The whites were only 25% around the time. The rest were Pacific Islanders, blacks, and other natives.

Fourth, Hawaii is one of the smallest states in the country and one of the least populated. However, it also has a very high population density, which means more people are occupying a certain square mile of land than other states.

Fifth, it is a state that has its own official language besides English. The Hawaiian language is extremely unique that despite trying to learn some of the words, I really could not properly spell or memorize them. Nevertheless, I always considered their tone and the overall language to be very pleasing to the ears. To say that the island is beautiful is actually an understatement. I sometimes think that when I am already old and I needed a good place to retire and be at peace, Hawaii will be one of my top most choices. The people were very gentle, kind, and friendly. The natural sceneries are incredibly divine, from the surfing waves of the beaches to the fertile valleys and lush rainforests, everything was just amazing. It has a long-standing tradition that remains to be practiced and respected even by the new generation. It is where I truly felt as if everyone cared about everyone.

## To the Gorgeous Island of Hawaii

I arrived in Hawaii during the summer, so it is expected that the population of tourists was at an all-time high. Fortunately I was able to secure a hotel room and booked a flight many months before I left, so I can travel on a budget.

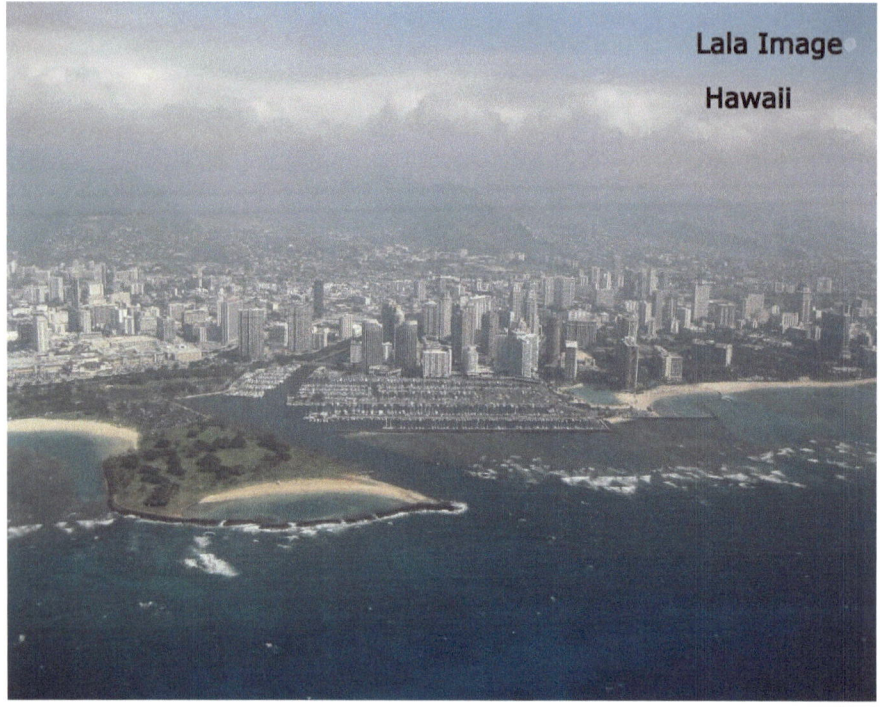

Hawaii has a lot of equally majestic islands, but considering my very limited funds, I had to make a choice and picked Honolulu simply because it is the state's capital and transport from the mainland to here will be much easier for me. I was also very excited to visit Waikiki.

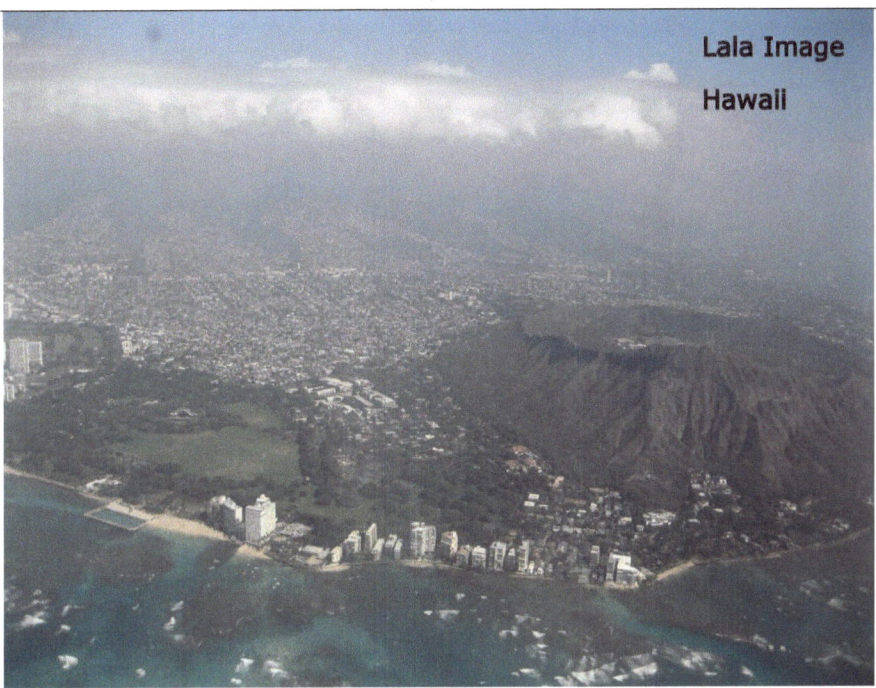

Lala Image

Hawaii

Waikiki is part of the Honolulu County, where the primary city is also Honolulu. It is well-known for its beaches and the waves. Trying to fulfill my desire, I booked a surfing lesson online. Immediately a day after my arrival, I met with the instructor and tried some techniques in the sand, especially when it comes to balancing on the board and going up the waters after falling. After an hour of initial training, we were then ready to ride the waves. It was insane! The experience was both nerve-racking, embarrassing, yet extremely rewarding. I fell more often than I stood. The only consolation was the fact that I was not the only one. My instructor was also very patient with me. I believe he was used to seeing most of his students failed.

Swimming and surfing can drain all your energy that a few minutes after arriving onshore, I gorged on sandwiches and a large glass of fruit shake in a nearby shack. It was heavenly.

Over the weekend, I went on a climb to Diamond Head (also known locally as Leahi). It is a very old crater with trails and stairs that lead you up to the area. If you are daring enough, you can also explore the underground tunnels and former military bunkers (as it used to serve as a lookout area). It was a convenient bus ride for a few minutes from the main Waikiki Beach.

In the afternoon, I joined a tour following a heritage trail around the neighborhood. We visited more than 15 of these sites. By the evening, I went back to the beach to listen to some feel-good live music and hang out with the locals and other tourists. It is as laid-back as you can get, and Hawaii, I realized, was just what I needed so that I can recharge myself and feel newer when I get back to work.

A few days before I left Hawaii, I changed my landscape from the beach to the land. I traveled to downtown Honolulu to visit the Museum of Art and Shangri-la and Queen Emma Summer Palace. I also took the time to pay tribute to the fallen soldiers during World War II by going to Pearl Harbor. More than a thousand died during the attack and which marked the beginning of the Second World War. The tour covered Pacific Aviation Museum and USS Arizona Memorial.

# Part 16

# Me and the Rest of the World

Aside from being able to see most of the United States, I was also privileged to visit a lot of international destinations — too many, in fact, my entire experiences in these places demand a different book.

However, just to give you some idea where I had been, let me talk about them in brief:

## Jamaica

Jamaica will always have a special place in my heart. It's where I was born and part of who I am. We don't have extensive nightlife or shopping districts as in the U.S., but we are proud of our beautiful lush natural resources. Some of the most well-known attractions are Blue Hole in Ocho Rios, Seven-Mile Beach, Rio Grande in Port Antonio, Mystic Mountain, White River, and Dolphin Cove. We have some of the most beautiful world-class golf courses perched high on a mountain and overlooking our crystal-clear blue waters. Transport in our country is extremely varied, and it's possible to commute through local taxis, buses, and trains.

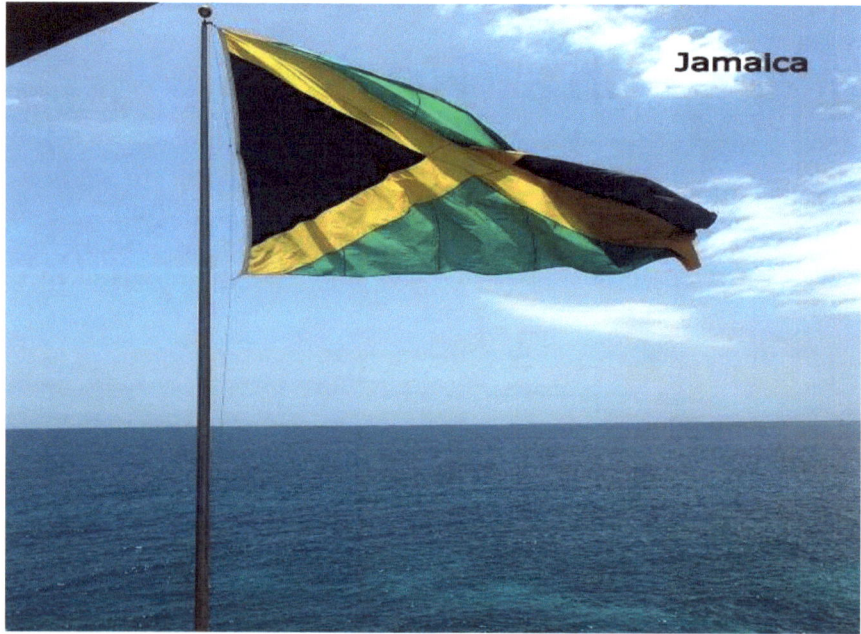

## Canada

Sharing a border with the United States, Canada is actually quite accessible. My friends and I decided to visit our neighbors up there and went to Ontario because we truly wanted to see the famous Niagara Falls. We enjoyed a thrilling ride in a Jet Boat Tour that took us along the same path taken by the War of 1812 soldiers, but heck, I couldn't remember the history anymore because I was so busy trying to stay alive! Despite that, I am so glad I did it because it helped me test my resolve for adventure. We also balanced the hair-raising ride with a fancy visit to the nearby Botanical Gardens.

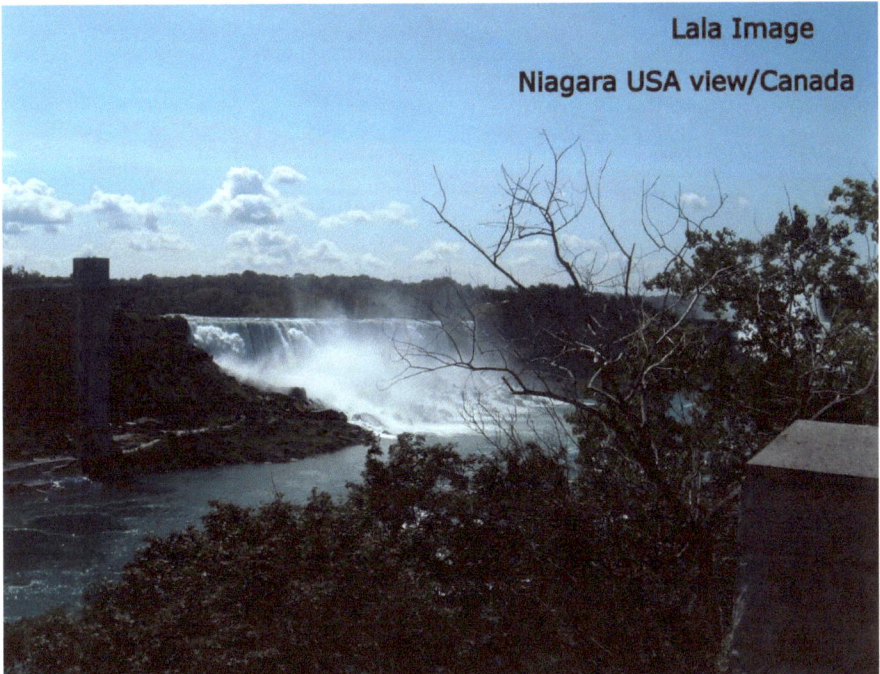

Lala Image

Niagara USA view/Canada

## Great Britain

Visiting all those museums, looking at Renaissance and 19th-century artworks in both public and private galleries, strolling along cemeteries and gardens that referenced the Victorian Era definitely encouraged me to go to Europe, especially Great Britain — and I did!

I stayed there for a few weeks, and around this time, I ended in London, Liverpool, Nottingham, Southampton, Leeds, and Leicester. Although quite expensive, I enjoyed a nice London cab, enjoyed walking tours especially around Nottingham, Southampton, and the alleys of London, watched a performance in West End, and of course rode the Tube. I stayed in a cozy bread and breakfast that served incredible tea every morning.

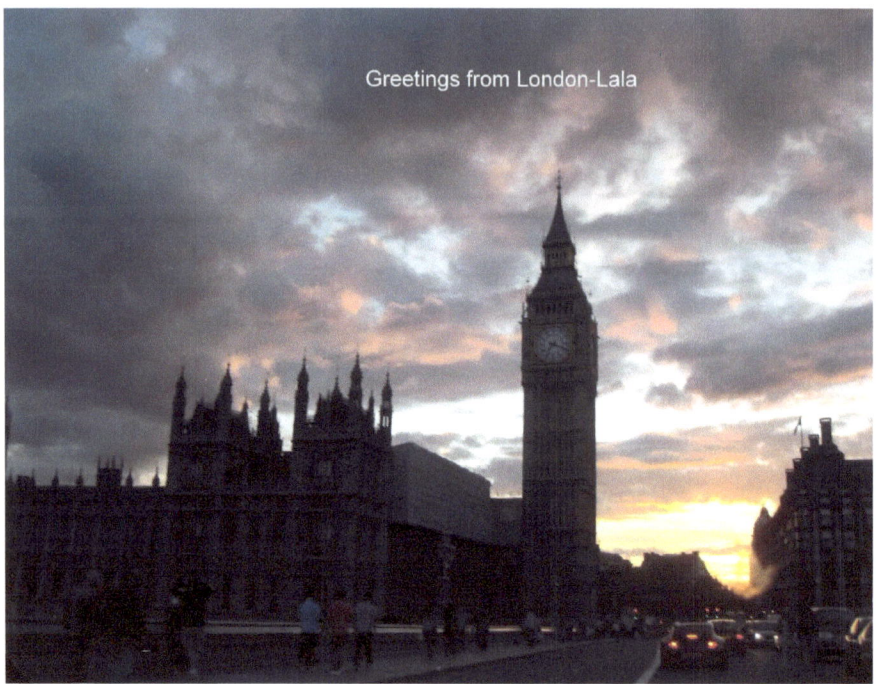

Greetings from London-Lala

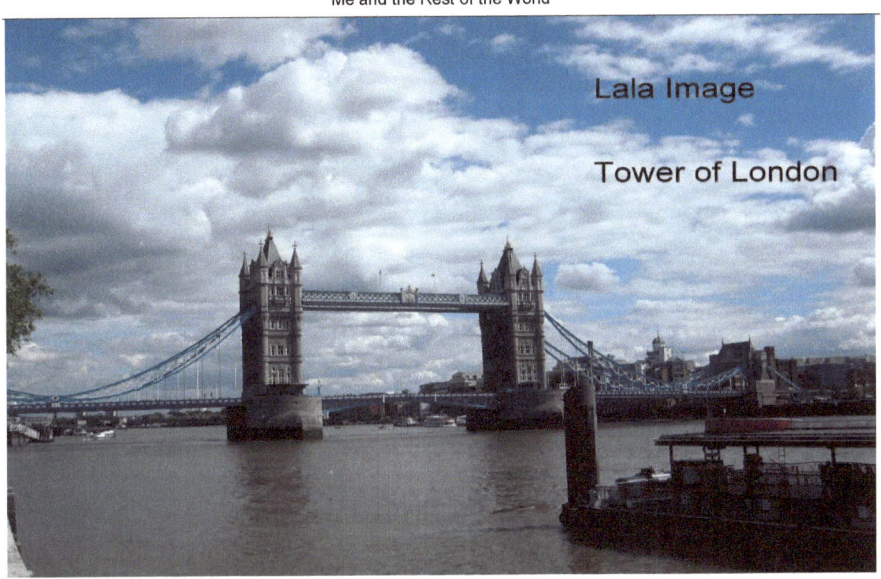

Lala Image

Tower of London

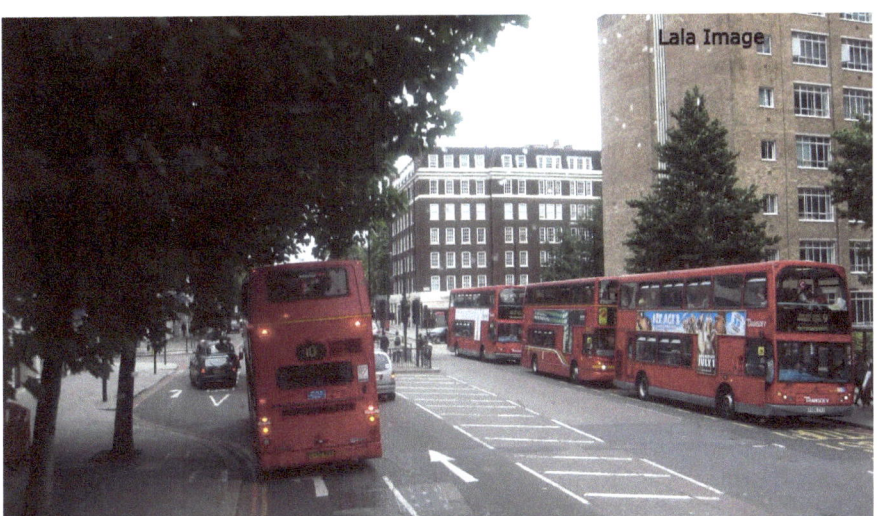

Lala Image

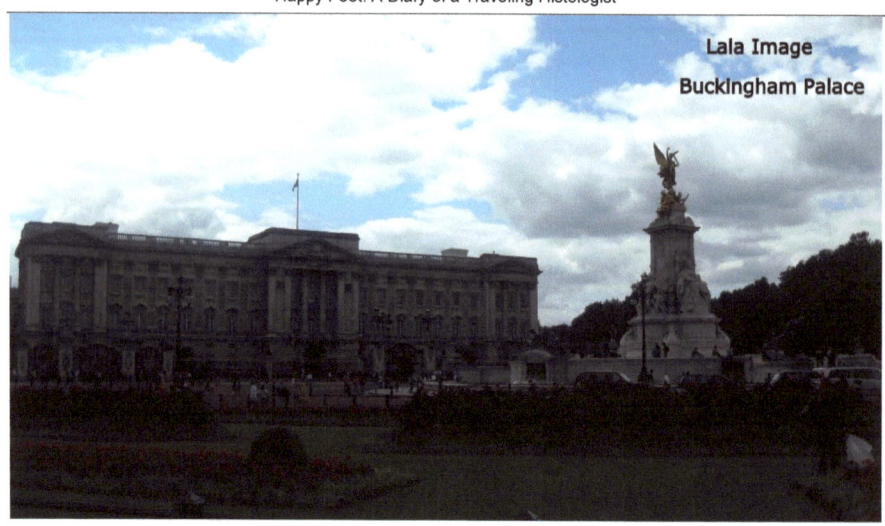

Lala Image

Buckingham Palace

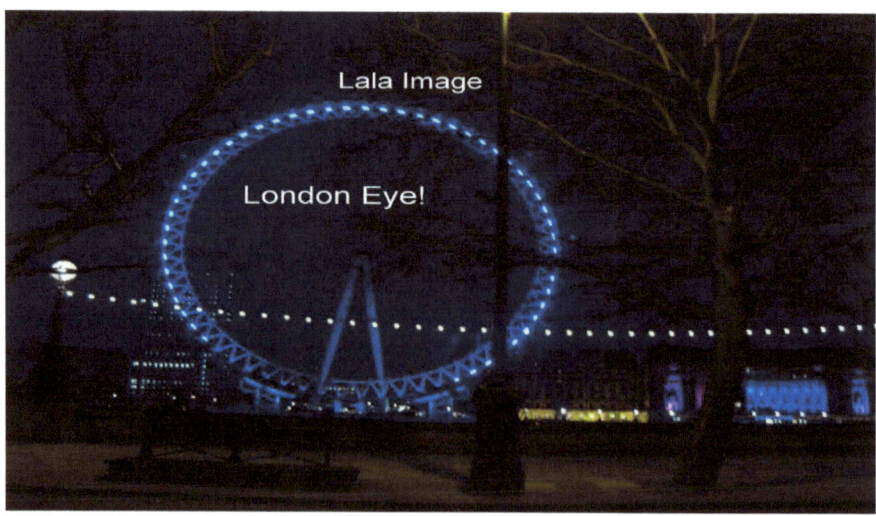

Lala Image

London Eye!

## Denmark

Since I was already in Europe, I continued backpacking, so from London, I moved to Denmark, specifically Copenhagen, its capital. It's incredible how the country is able to combine work and play so effortlessly. Men in suits hop on their bike to and from work. They always took the time to relax and drink their beers or walk along the parks. Since I wanted to enjoy like the locals did, I rented a bike during the duration of my stay. I checked out museums like National Museum of Denmark, Rosenborg Castle, and Church of Our Lady. I was amazed by the Statue of the Little Mermaid and ogled at the unique-looking buildings in the metro.

## Sweden

After my stay in Denmark, I hopped on a train that took me to Sweden, which was just as charming as Denmark and Great Britain. I went to Stockholm and Malmo. Although I definitely had a lot of fun checking out the old architecture and the remnants of the ancient Scandinavians, I was more interested in food. Cafes are all over the place, usually serving coffee paired with a sweet treat. It's very common among people here to take their time alone or with company. One of the locals I befriended invited me on a beer-drinking spree on a boat! In Malmo, I dined on eel, dairy, and other local produce.

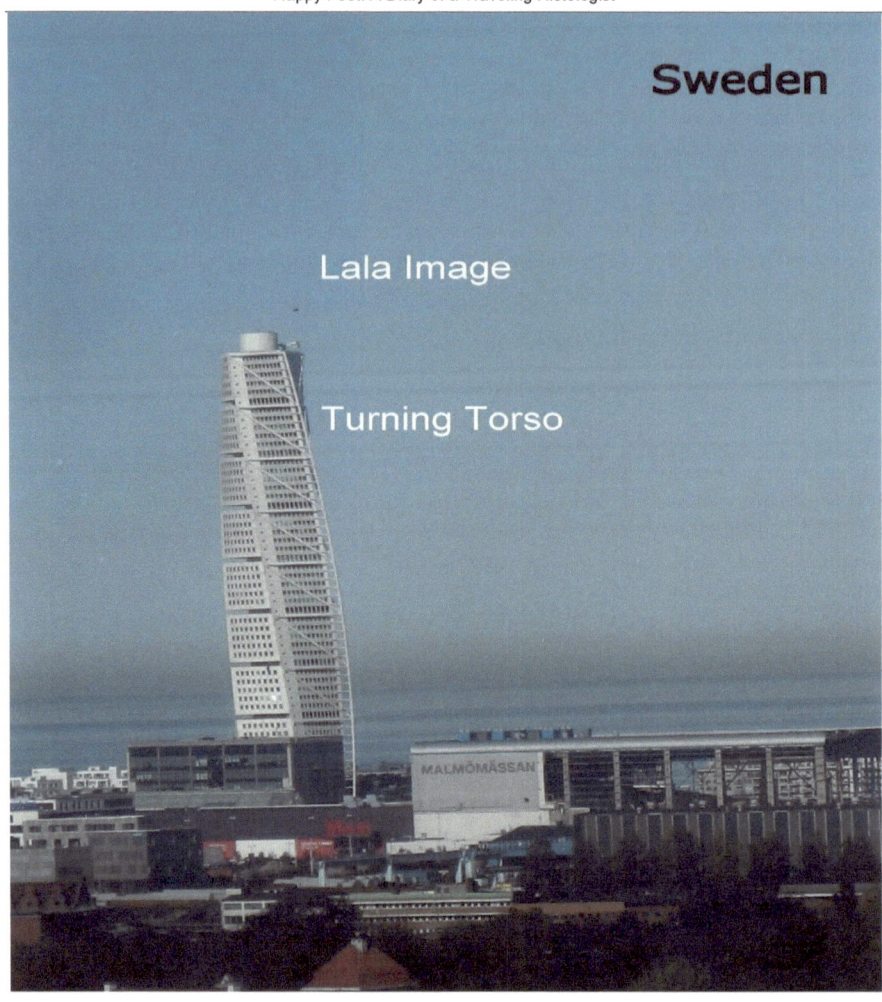

Sweden

Lala Image

Turning Torso

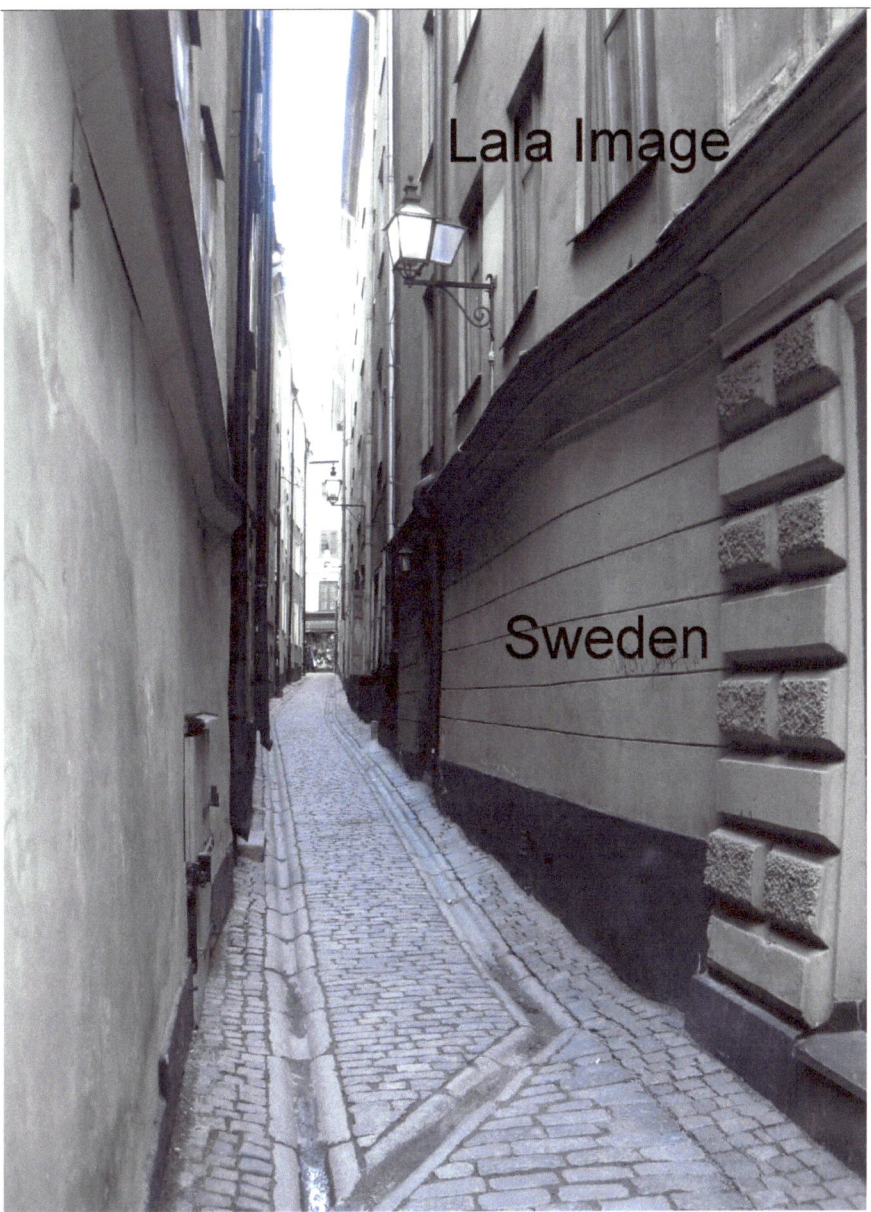

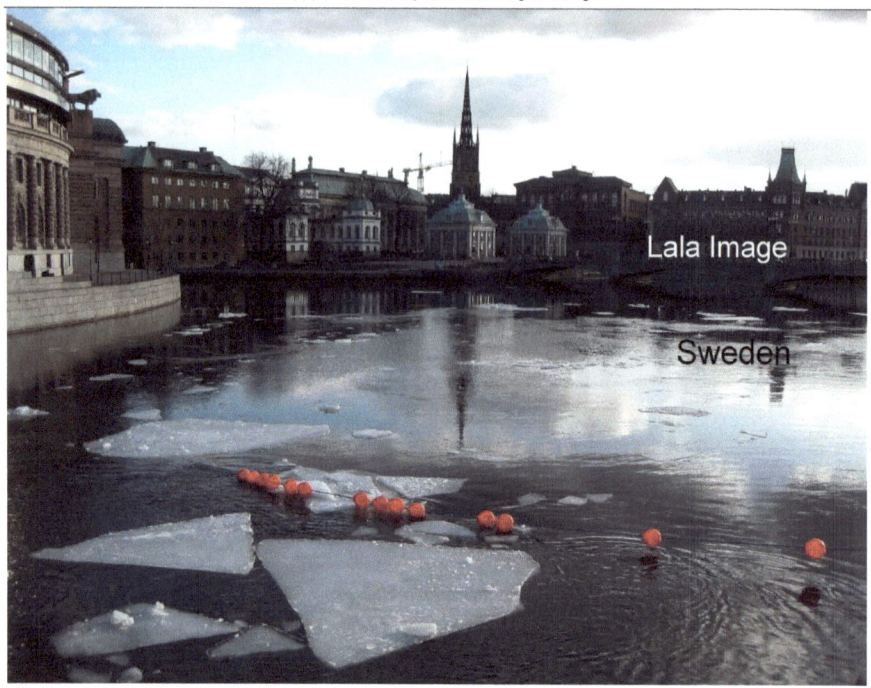

## Switzerland

I have to admit that my first impression of Switzerland was chocolates, but that was *before* I arrived there. It turns out that it offers more than the delectable treat. Hiking is a very popular activity here, thanks to its scenic mountains and natural landscapes like Swiss National Park, as well as retreats in villages surrounded by those lush forests and tall mountains. In Geneva, I explored Yvette de Marseilles, L'Adresee, and Old Town. Mini train tours afforded me to see some very interesting parts of the city in a short amount of time.

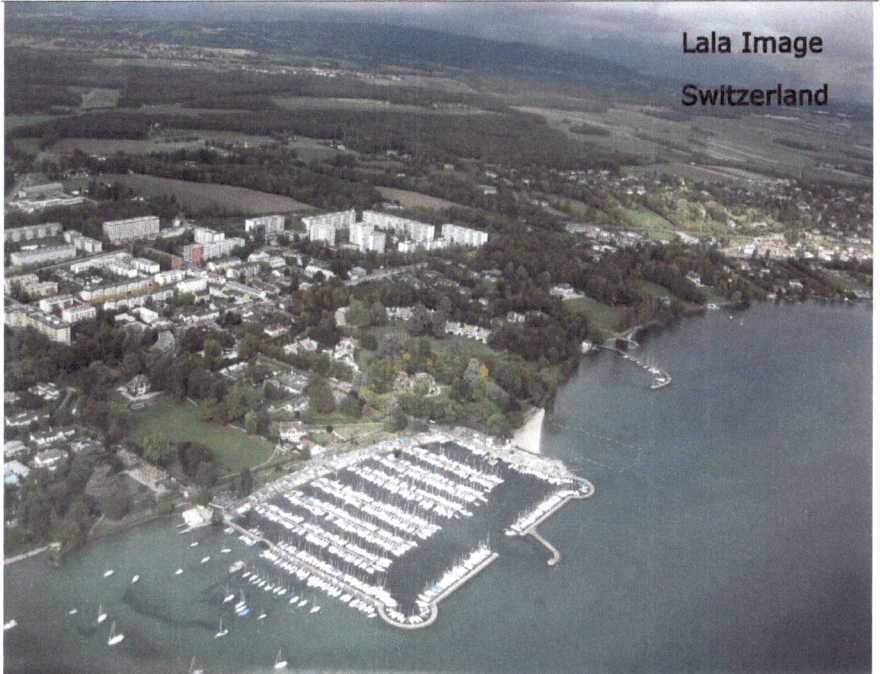

Lala Image
Switzerland

## Amsterdam

I saw *Fault in Our Stars* a couple of days ago and I immediately remembered my short but memorable trip to Amsterdam. Traveling was very convenient because they have trams, metro lines, and even scooters and bicycles that you can rent for a very cheap price. Since I tried bicycles before, I chose scooters that time. Amsterdam looks like a very large open museum since most of the buildings are considered historical sites. The Canal Ring allowed me to see the city in a boat—much like when you're in Venice, Italy.

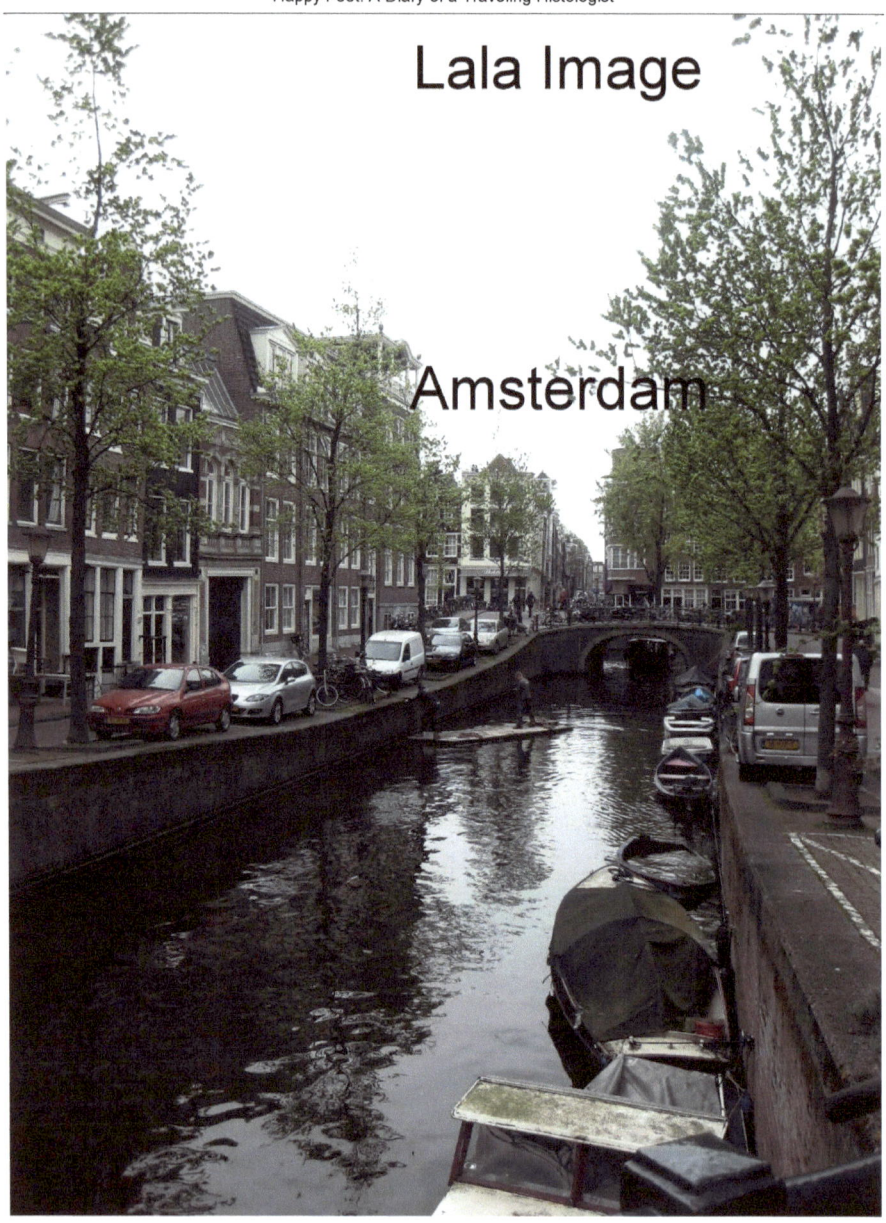

Lala Image

Amsterdam

## France

France is often called the city that never sleeps or the most romantic place in the entire world. I just think it's friendly to tourists. It's a very well-planned country and its beauty goes past famous cities and places like Paris and St. Tropez. I stayed for a bit in Calais, Dover, Castellane, Canne, Marseille, Monaco, Monte-Carlo, and Brignoles. From wineries and vineyards to UNESCO World Heritage Sites, the Eiffel Tower, countless museums and galleries, and lots of pastries, I can safely say that France deserves to be one of the top tourist destinations in the world.

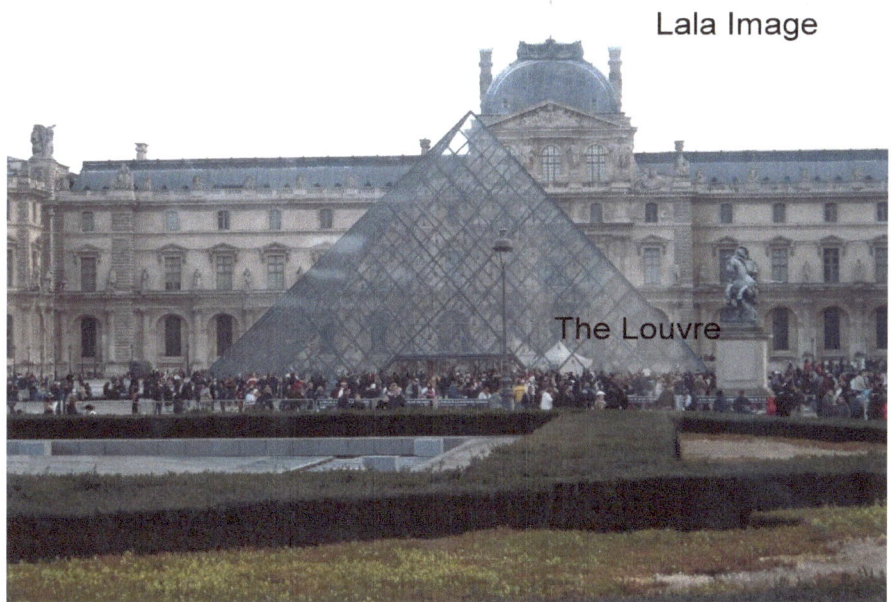

Lala Image

The Louvre

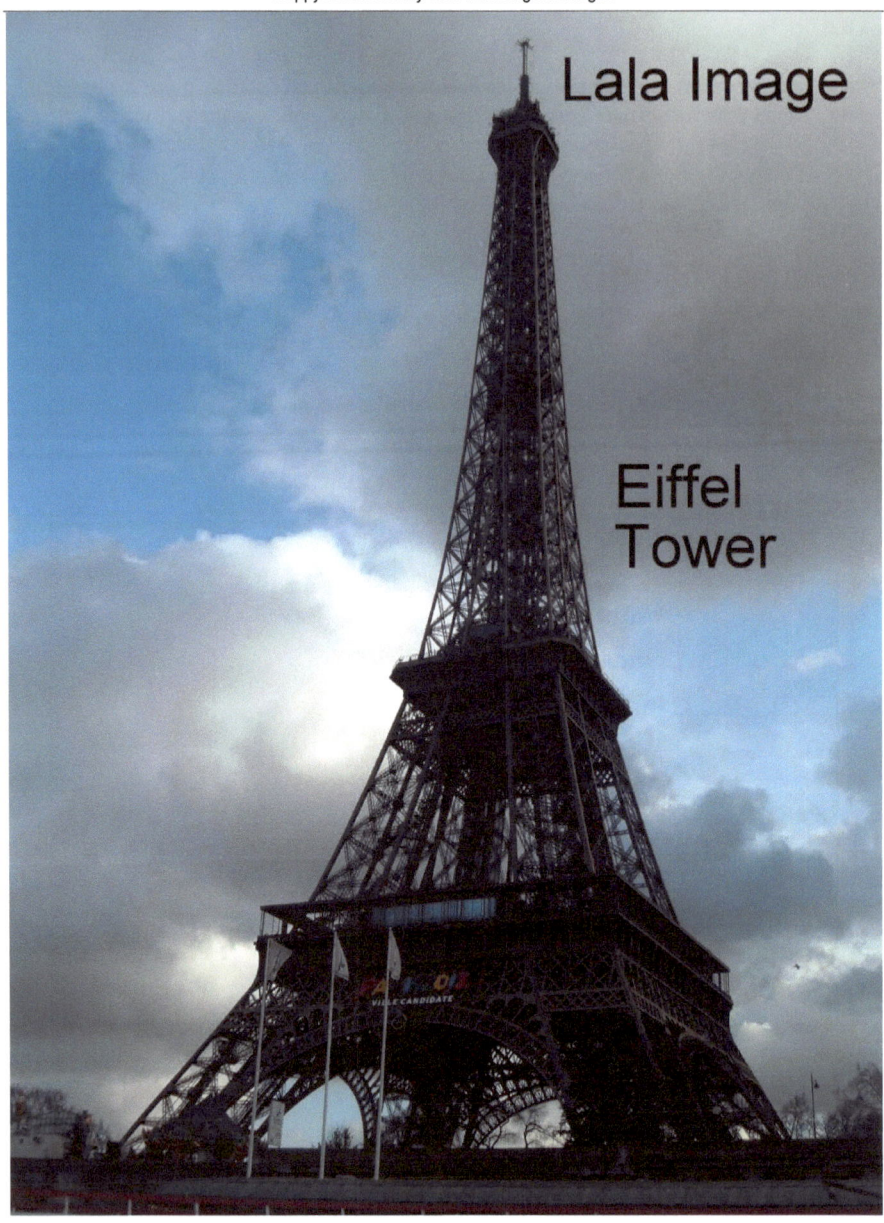

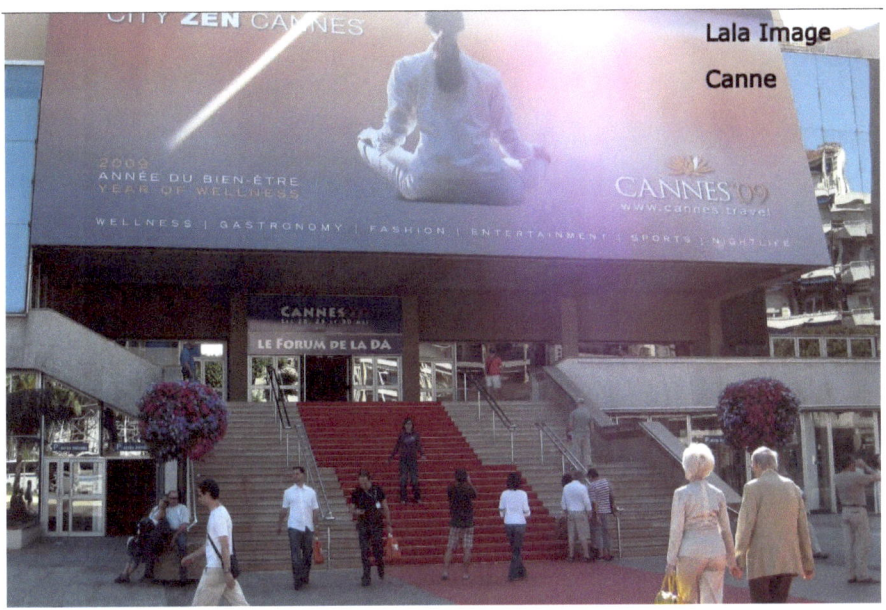

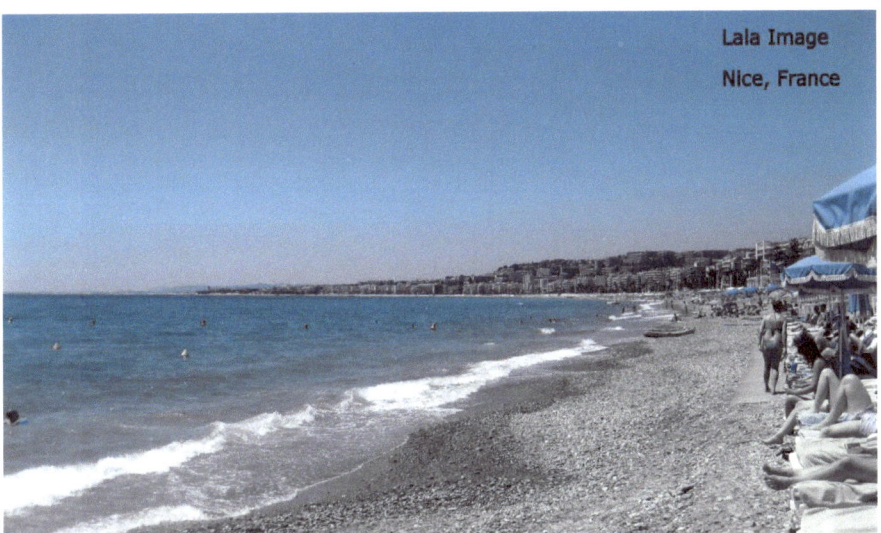

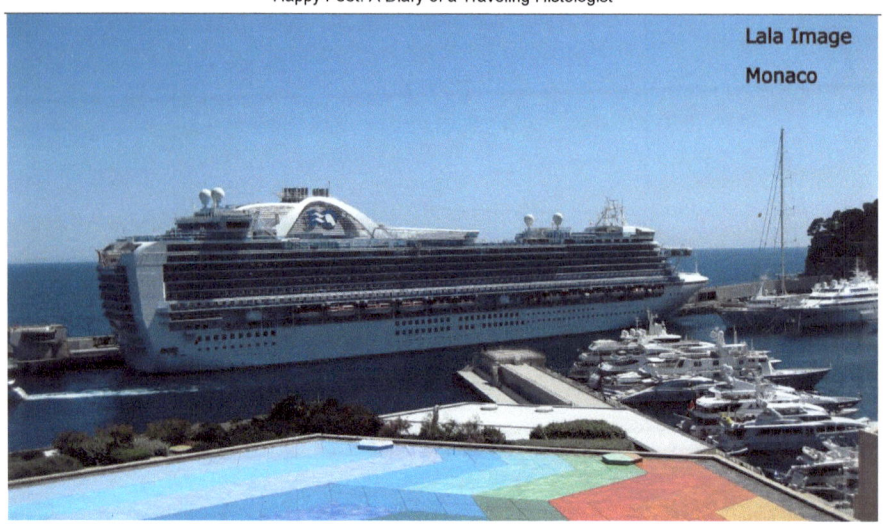

Lala Image
Monaco

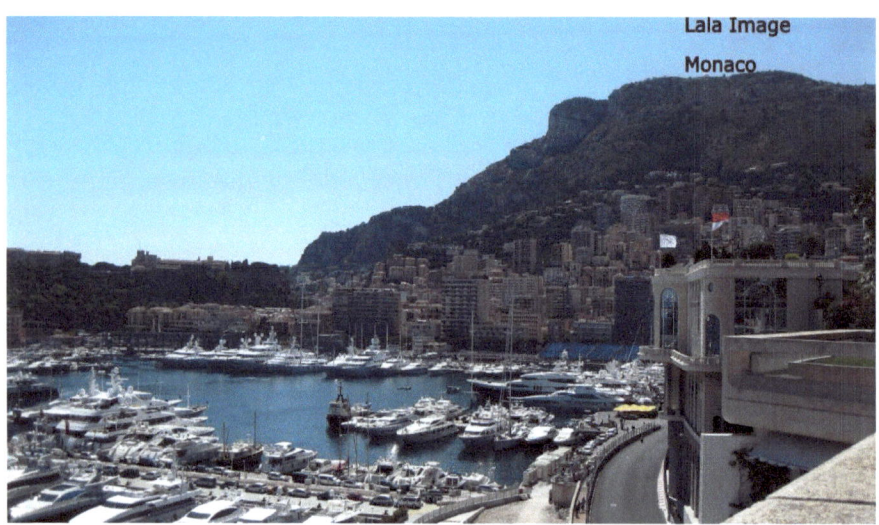

Lala Image
Monaco

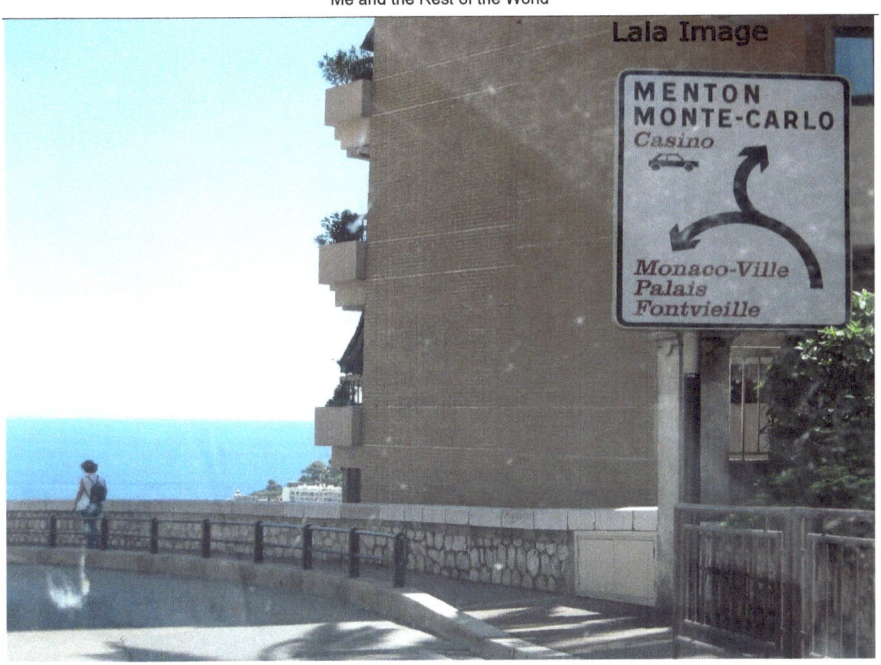

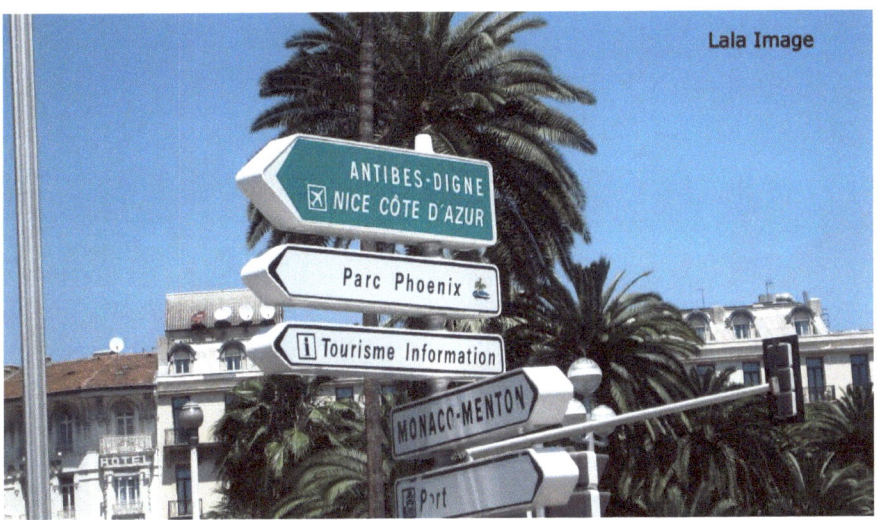

## The UAE

Dubai is a very expensive city, so you really have to prepare for it, but if you simply do your research well and plan ahead, it's manageable for every budget traveler. Traveling around the city is convenient with the Metro, which is its extensive and modern railway system, although taxis are still aplenty. The city is actually divided into two: Old and New. Where you should go depends on your goal. If you want to see more historic sites, then Old is your choice. Meanwhile, if you want to experience the future of Dubai and even that of other competitive cities, I highly recommend the New Dubai, which includes the very tall structures of Burj Al-Khalifa and Dubai Marina.

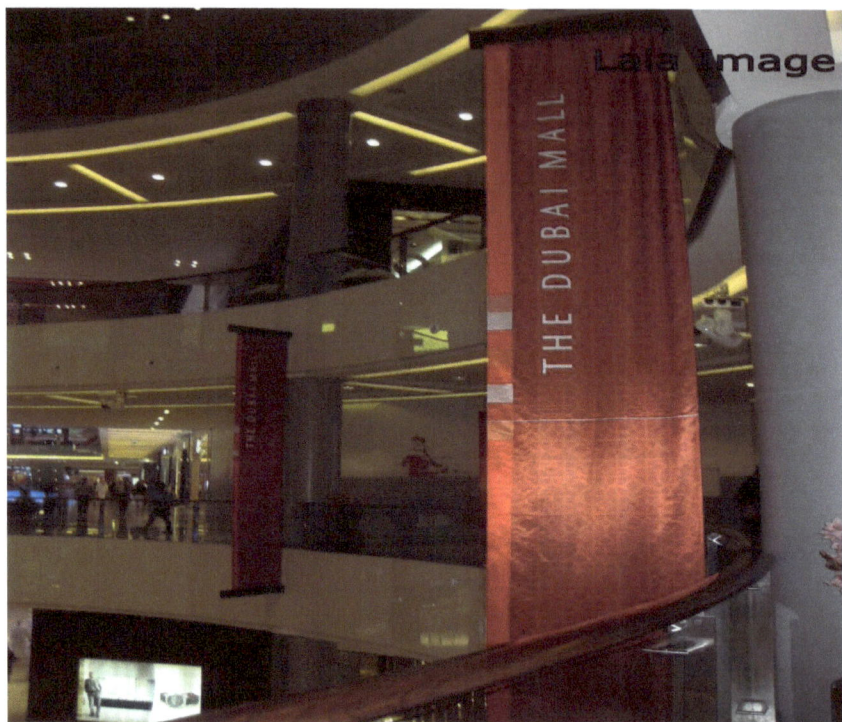

## Africa

For many decades, Africa has obtained an ill reputation especially when it comes to travelers (particularly, women). I have to be honest that I was quite apprehensive to take on the journey. I did my research and found out that, although some places still have to be avoided at all costs, a good number are great for all types of tourists. My ultimate goal was to visit Zanzibar, but en route, I stopped for two days in Dar Es Salaam. I wanted to ride the *dala-dala* but, I deemed it dangerous, so I took a taxi instead. Around the city, I simply walked around its market selling a variety of produce and souvenirs such as Tinga-Tinga paintings.

When I got to Zanzibar, I joined a walking tour around Stone Town and a spice tour in Zanzibar Island.

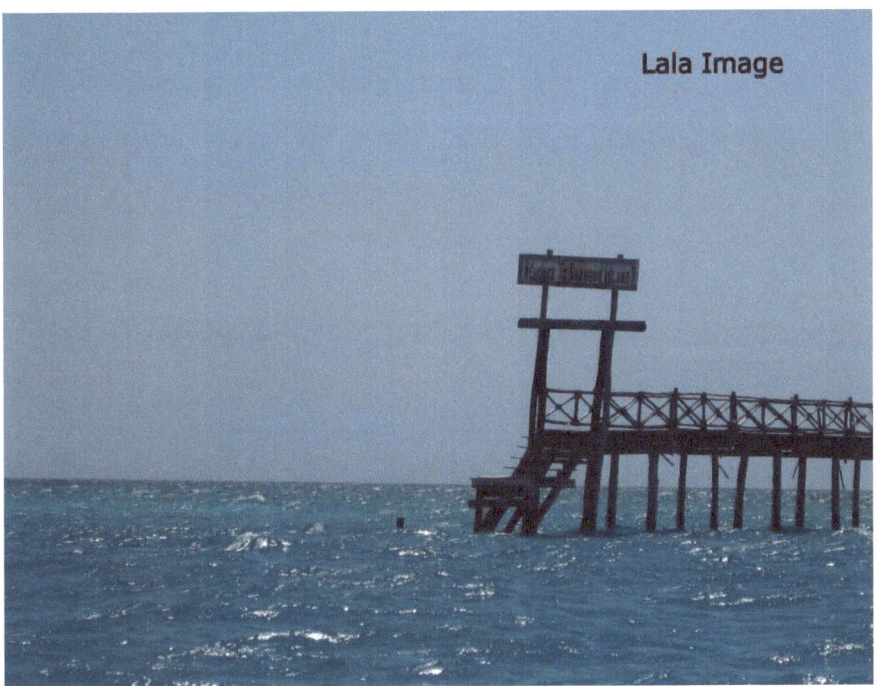

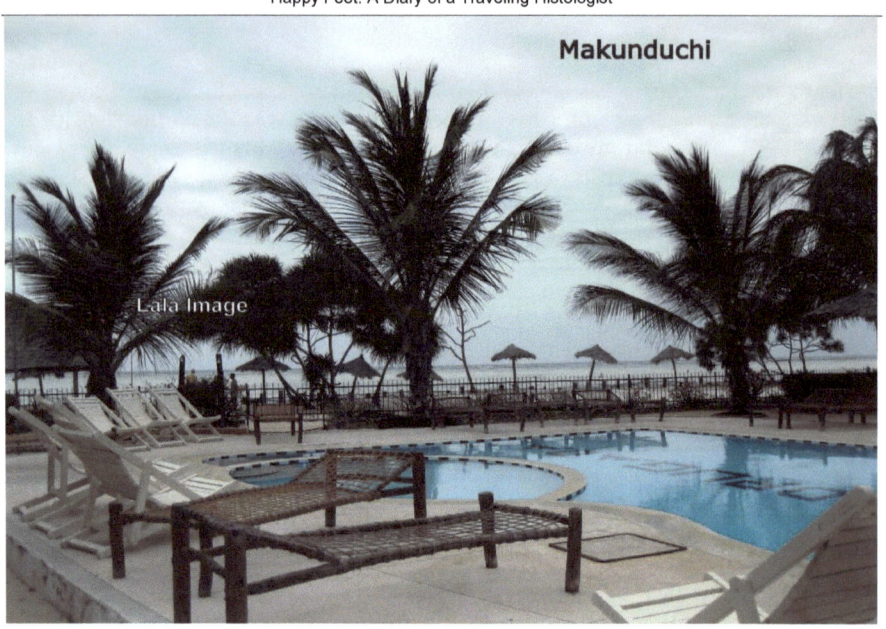

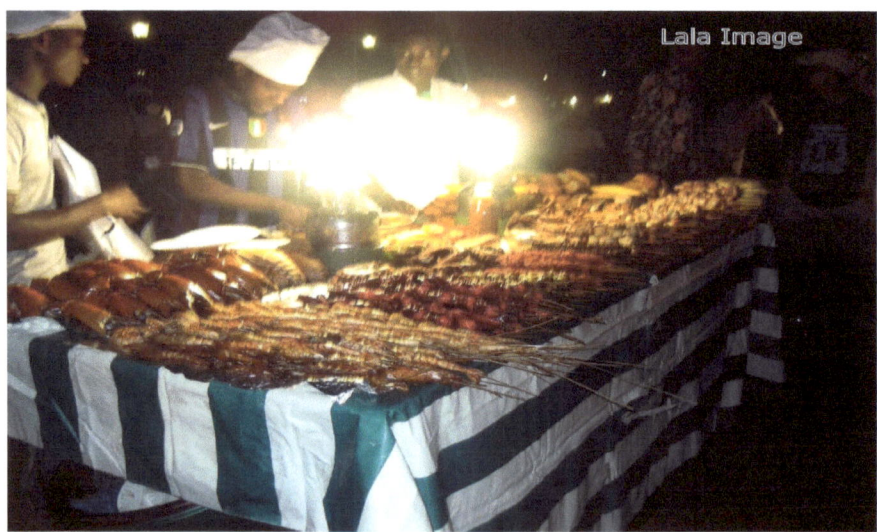

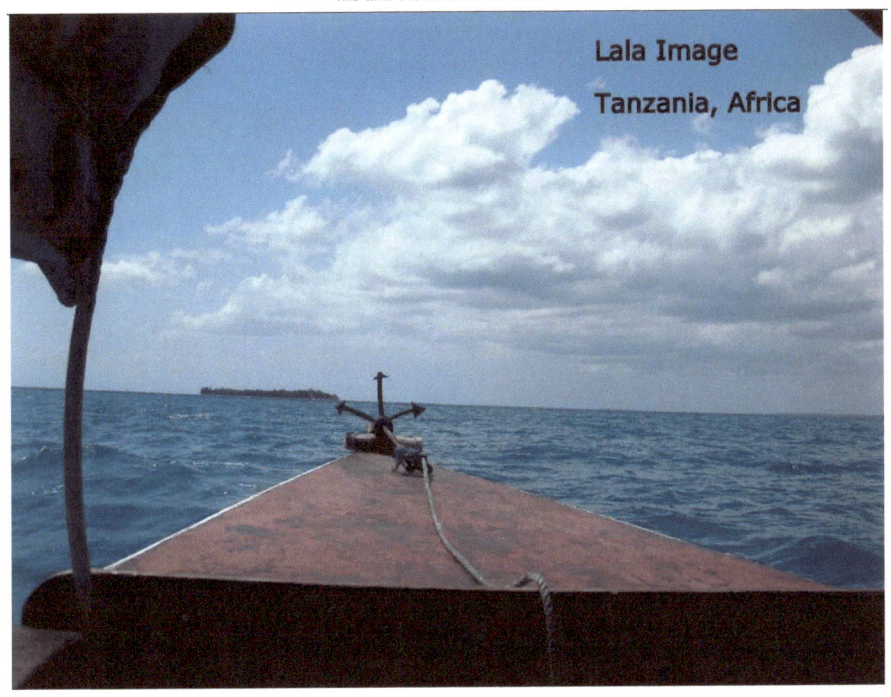

Lala Image
Tanzania, Africa

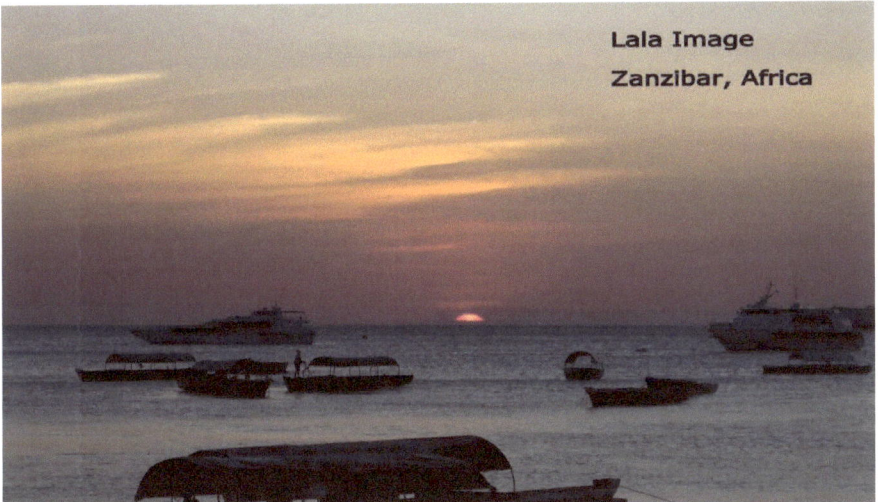

Lala Image
Zanzibar, Africa

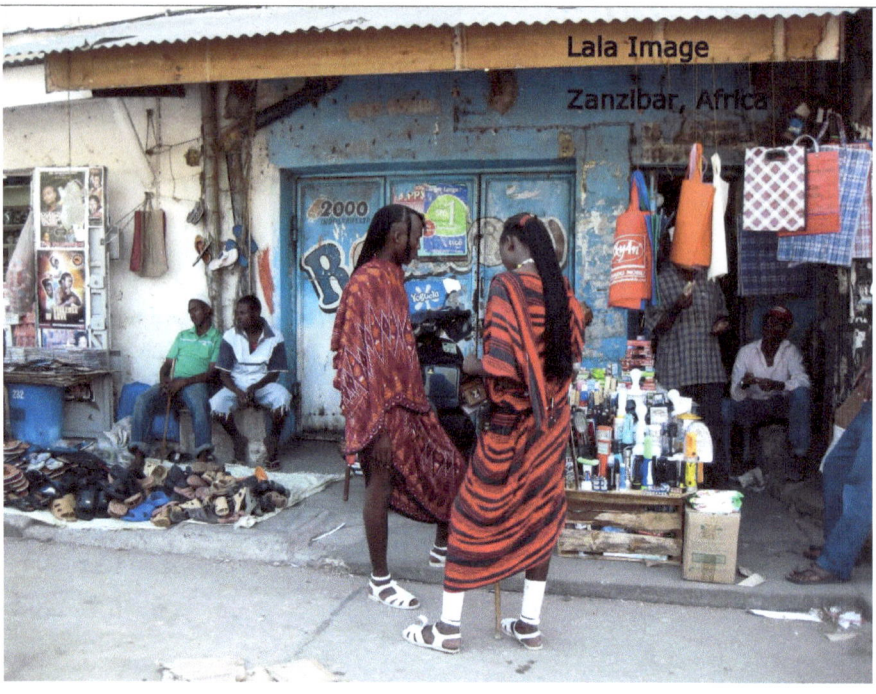

# Closing

I have found traveling exciting and rewarding. It has allowed me to forge new friendships along the way. The memories are forever imprinted within your mind. I have been able to work when I want, take time off when desired, and maintain a good lifestyle. Not bad! The saga continues on to the travel job.

Isaiah 60:1 KJV Arise, shine; for thy light is come…Blessings!

## Resources

**Airlines:**
American Airlines www.aa.com
AirTran www.airtran.com
British Airways www.ba.com
Delta www.delta.com
JetBlue www.jetblue.com
RyanAir www.ryanair.com
Southwest www.southwest.com
Spirit www.spiritairlines.com
United www.united.com
Virgin Atlantic Airways www.virgin-atlantic.com

**Rental Cars:**
Avis www.avis.com
Hertz www.hertz.com
Alamo  www.alamo.com
National www.nationalcar.com
Budget www.budget.com
Thrifty www.thrifty.com
Enterprise www.enterprise.com

**Websites:**
American Society for Clinical Pathology Board of Certification (BOC) www. ascp.org
National Society for Histotechnology www.nsh.org

**Books:**
Living up to Life www.leica-microsystems.com
Histotechnology A Self-Assessment Workbook
Board of Registry Study Guide Practice Questions for the Histotechology Examinations
www.ascp.org

**Magazines :**
Lab Medicine, The Journal for Medical laboratory professionals www.labmedicine.com

**Notes**

www.ingramcontent.com/pod-product-compliance
Lightning Source LLC
Chambersburg PA
CBHW040808200526

45159CB00022B/59